PRACTICING
LIBERATION
WORKBOOK

RADICAL TOOLS FOR GRASSROOTS ACTIVISTS,
COMMUNITY LEADERS, TEACHERS, AND CARETAKERS
WORKING TOWARD SOCIAL JUSTICE

PRACTICING LIBERATION WORKBOOK

Written and edited by Hala Khouri, Tessa Hicks Peterson, and Keely Nguyễn

WITH CONTRIBUTIONS FROM JACOBY BALLARD, BELOVED COMMUNITIES
NETWORK, LESLIE BOOKER, SCARLETT DUARTE, KAZU HAGA, HAIZE HAWKE,
KERRI KELLY, MOBIUS, AND SUSY ZEPEDA

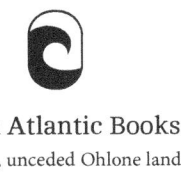

North Atlantic Books
Huichin, unceded Ohlone land
Berkeley, California

Published by
North Atlantic Books
Huichin, unceded Ohlone land
Berkeley, California

Printed in Canada

Cover art and design by Amanda Weiss
Book design by Happenstance Type-O-Rama

Practicing Liberation Workbook: Radical Tools for Grassroots Activists, Community Leaders, Teachers, and Caretakers Working Toward Social Justice is sponsored and published by North Atlantic Books, an educational nonprofit based in the unceded Ohlone land Huichin (Berkeley, CA) that collaborates with partners to develop cross-cultural perspectives; nurture holistic views of art, science, the humanities, and healing; and seed personal and global transformation by publishing work on the relationship of body, spirit, and nature.

North Atlantic Books's publications are distributed to the US trade and internationally by Penguin Random House Publisher Services. For further information visit our website at www.northatlanticbooks.com.

Library of Congress Cataloging-in-Publication Data

Names: Khouri, Hala, author. | Peterson, Tessa Hicks, author. | Nguyen, Keely, author.
Title: Practicing liberation workbook : radical tools for grassroots activists, community leaders, teachers, and caretakers working toward social justice / by Hala Khouri, Tessa Hicks Peterson, and Keely Nguyen.
Description: Berkeley, CA : North Atlantic Books, [2024] | Includes bibliographical references.
Identifiers: LCCN 2023050116 (print) | LCCN 2023050117 (ebook) | ISBN 9798889840688 (trade paperback) | ISBN 9798389840695 (ebook)
Subjects: LCSH: Social justice. | Social change. | Community development. | Psychic trauma. | Social reformers—Mental health. | Stress (Psychology).
Classification: LCC HM671 .H53 2024 (print) | LCC HM671 (ebook) | DDC 303.3/72—dc23/eng/20231106
LC record available at https://lccn.loc.gov/2023050116
LC ebook record available at https://lccn.loc.gov/2023050117

1 2 3 4 5 6 7 8 9 MARQUIS 23 27 26 25 24

North Atlantic Books is committed to the protection of our environment. We print on recycled paper whenever possible and partner with printers who strive to use environmentally responsible practices.

This book is dedicated to those we are most intimately accountable to: our beloved blood and chosen families, our ancestors, known and unknown, and our future descendants. It is also dedicated to the many young people, elders, community organizers, artists, healers, colleagues, comrades, and collaborators we have been blessed to work with in our communities, grassroots collectives, and larger institutions for change. We are grateful to all those who have generously shared their wisdom and practices of liberation with us, and who have asked us to pay it forward. This is for you (and you, and you . . .).

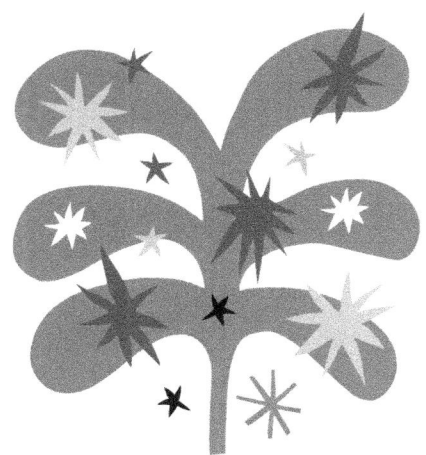

CONTENTS

PART II COMMUNITY BUILDING AND CONNECTION

PART III COLLECTIVE IMAGINING

ACKNOWLEDGMENTS

This workbook (and the anthology inspiring it) draws greatly from the work of so many. The influences are far and wide, from academic scholars in psychology, education, critical theory, and cultural studies to elders and mentors from spiritual traditions, organizations, and movement spaces we have been a part of. We are grateful to bring practices to these pages that we have learned in many spaces over many decades, and hope that we have honored them well. We are cognizant in particular that in recent years, calls for community care and emergent strategies have grown strongly in our circles of frontline changemakers, healers, and scholars desiring more transformative practices to sustain individuals and movements. We want to name and uplift healing justice, which has emerged within the last twenty years as a powerful collective care movement to address generational trauma and oppression and radically reimagine collective care, safety, accountability, and healing as part of liberatory political strategy and practice. Healing justice emerged formally in 2006 through Kindred Southern Healing Justice Collective, alongside other directly impacted feminist activists and healers who survive trauma and oppression by drawing on embodied liberatory practices. With strong roots in anticapitalism, abolition, and Black feminism, this framework is integral to paradigm shifts in organizations and communities yearning for more roadmaps that are justice oriented, healing centered, and community led. Healing justice recognizes the need for changemaking work to weave together ancestral wisdom traditions of healing and knowledge around community care and repair with critical imaginings of change that do not reproduce systemic -isms and interpersonal harm. We are grateful to the many BIPOC feminist organizers and scholar-activists across space and time that have advanced this movement.

We also acknowledge the diverse ancestors of our writing collective and hope we are doing justice to their dreams of the future. Likewise, we hope to do justice to our future descendants, who desperately need us to practice liberation, community care, and healing justice now so that they may have a thriving future to be born into. We recognize our accountability to them both, as well as to the earth and the Indigenous communities who seeded original restorative practices and community care long before this country was colonized. Further, we respectfully acknowledge and are indebted to the labor of the multitudes who have been forced onto this land and continue to work in the shadows for our collective benefit; this includes enslaved people and refugee- and immigrant-settlers, many of whom have been coerced to this country by militarism, imperialism, and displacement. We also understand that acknowledgment alone is insufficient to address and begin to repair the historic and ongoing harm caused by colonialism, white supremacy, and centuries of attempted genocide. We hope this work plays one small part in the larger work of reparations and community care by way of gifting back knowledges that advance healing justice to more and more of us who inhabit this fragile planet, as well as gifting back actual dollars from the residuals of this book toward funds for Indigenous rematriation.

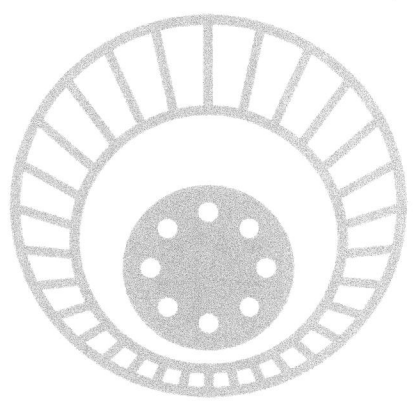

INTRODUCTION

This workbook is a love letter, a journal, and a guide for all those who work tirelessly for well-being and justice against a backdrop of conditions that cause harm to so many. This book is for anyone working toward healing, uplifting, and transforming our world. It is for grassroots activists, community organizers, educators, and mental health workers; it is for first responders, medical professionals, parents, and caretakers. We call you changemakers. And, we want you to be well. We need you to be well. We, too, are changemakers and know how hard it is to fully embody the well-being that is our birthright and that we are fighting for in the world. Well-being and liberation can feel unattainable when we are faced with suffering and injustice as well as impossible workloads inside of systems that don't serve us. Yet, we are hopeful and fully dedicated to transforming our systems from the inside out and creating realities inside our individual and collective bodies that reflect what is possible. We (the collective who contributed to this workbook) have crafted this offering to support others who want to join us in this ancient and beautiful struggle.

Changemakers everywhere are facing high levels of stress, which often lead to burnout and health challenges on an individual level, and conflict, high turnover, and even abuse at an organizational level. Many of us are dealing with systemic trauma—violence, inequity, and oppression that is perpetuated on structural and institutional levels inside of systems of education, healthcare, law, finance, public policy, and beyond. These systems often privilege certain individuals and communities and exclude, disregard, or harm others. This results in what we call the *trauma of injustice*, stemming from racism, ableism, sexism, transphobia, heterosexism, classism, ageism, xenophobia, religious bigotry, and any other form of identity-based oppression.

Because of this we need practices to help us cope and heal, not just so we can be well ourselves, but so we can continue the important work of challenging inequity and a culture that ranks our worth and pits our needs against each other. Radical care for ourselves and our community expands the capacity of individuals, organizations, and collectives to build cultures of justice, care, and mutuality together, with a rippling impact in the rest of the world.

Most changemakers today have tremendous skills and practices for personal and organizational resiliency in the face of the tyranny of the world. But, what if the tyranny of exhaustion and stress is partially self-imposed and actually limiting the vision of the world we want? What if we could integrate new ideas, tools, and practices into our personal and collective lives that would elevate commitments to caring for ourselves and our communities and translate into more sustainable ways in which our organizations and movements could operate? What if we discovered that slowing down to take care, to invest in relationships, to put the values of community liberation and wellness into our daily work practices and structures actually allows us to feel better and more interconnected as we do the work of re-creating a better world? What if we created the world we want in the one we have and even felt joy, connection, and sustainability in the process of that hard work of change? What if the work itself felt life-giving and restorative rather than draining and conflictual?

Many before us have emphasized the importance of connecting changemaking work to radical healing practices. "Radical" means going to the root, to the spirit of the matter. Indigenous communities and ancient wisdom traditions throughout the world have long held at the root of their values the interconnectedness of mind, body, and spirit and of individuals, communities, and ecosystems. The models for regenerative and restorative practices that we desperately need today are as old as—and directly connected to—our impulse to repair the world. Thus, what we need is the very knowledge that we hold in our bones, in our ancestral memories, in histories both abandoned and stolen. What we offer here are vehicles for *re-membering*—that is, bringing the parts of such knowing and communal practicing back together, with the added value of what new science, consciousness, and traditions can bring to a (re)mix that will deepen and expand strategies to sustain ourselves in the world we live in today.

Often, the impact of systemic oppression and injustice can keep us in survival mode— constantly putting out fires and fighting for basic rights. This can make it feel impossible to have space to imagine what we want because all of our energy is going to dealing with the impacts of what we don't want. This is one aspect of the trauma of injustice—it can block our capacity to dream and imagine and keep us stuck in reactivity and crisis. When we center healing in our work, it can challenge and disrupt the ways we've become so accustomed to fighting that we get stuck, and even unconsciously attached to the fight. When we center healing, our work can become generative rather than just reactive. This allows us to respond to both harm and stress in a more generative way and envision and work toward the radical transformation of our systems. This requires us to be flexible and agile so we can move from crisis and urgent matters into spaces to connect and envision long-term solutions to the problems we are facing. The healing process can help us transform tendencies rooted in trauma and survival into more life-affirming traits that support us to move beyond surviving, to thriving.

When we speak of thriving, we speak here of all the things humans require in order to have our needs met, and to be safe, connected with, cared for, and well. Critical wellness is more than some singular notion of what is healthy; it does not set up a hierarchy of value on who is most fit, strong, and well or what it means to be those things for different bodies—which, in fact, excludes those who are unable to reach society's idealized notions of "health" due to any number of personal, political, economic, and cultural factors. We believe well-being is a state that enables us to integrate everything we know in our bones with what we feel in our hearts, with the awe and wisdom that exist in our spirits, with what our lived experiences tell us about who we are and what the world has to offer. This workbook aims to give readers practices and strategies to be well together; to thrive, heal, connect, and activate transformation on individual, collective, and organizational levels.

This workbook was inspired by our accompanying anthology on healing justice entitled *Practicing Liberation: Transformative Strategies for Collective Healing and Systems Change.*[1] Our hope is that this workbook is an accessible, user-friendly guide for anyone working in their communities or inside of organizations through activism, education, healing, mental health, community organizing, policy reform, fiscal or legal support, art, music, and so on. We imagine this may be especially helpful for changemakers in organizations that want their practices to support building a culture of care inside their walls so that they can contribute toward realizing this goal in the rest of the world. You may be an executive director, staff person, board member, community organizer, educator, or mental health worker. Or maybe you are a grassroots visionary finding unique and beautiful ways to work toward justice. Whatever kind of changemaker you are, this workbook is for you.

This workbook is divided into three parts. The first is about the personal work of self-regulation, self-awareness, and self-care that is foundational to building strong communities that are able to imagine and create new realities together. The second part offers practices to inspire and support groups of people working together toward changemaking goals in ways that are authentic, meaningful, values-aligned, sustainable, and creative. The last part invites us into imagining a more just and free world and gives us tools for mapping our way there.

It's important for individuals and organizations to work at all levels of inquiry and practice offered here; they are mutually supporting and part of a larger paradigm of healing justice commitments. This paradigm situates individual healing inside of interpersonal healing, which are both part of systemic change. The three are intertwined and interconnected and cannot be fully realized on their own (see the Theory of Change below). That said, at different times certain sections may be more relevant to the specific situations and circumstances you and those you work with find yourselves in. So, feel free to start with the practices that are most relevant and needed, but don't ignore or disregard those that you think you don't need—they may have more to offer than you realize! We must practice self-regulation, for example, to sustain ourselves to be of service in times of stress and suffering; we must practice good communication for collective care and organizational health; and we need critical self-awareness if we are going to be in community together in a way that doesn't reproduce the harms of dominant culture. All components are interconnected, just like the thread that weaves well-being and social change together.

THEORY OF CHANGE

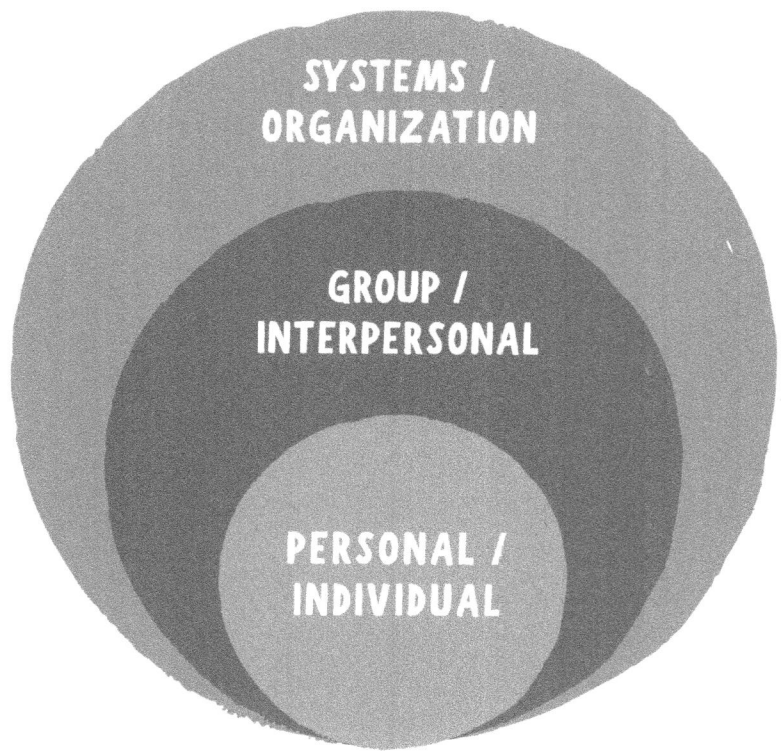

Many people contributed their words and practices to this workbook. In an effort to preserve and honor their language and framing, we are weaving their voices in as a tapestry. Rather than trying to create one uniform tone or voice, as editors, we want to honor the multiplicity of voices that are a part of our collective, which mirror, in many ways, the diverse voices that are part of our world's changemaking organizations and movements. Thus, you will see that while most sections were written or adapted by the editors, some are attributed to different collaborators who contributed to this offering. You might even find that some practices here are ones that you have done before, as many circulate among organizations and movements over time.

We want to also specifically acknowledge that many of the practices shared here have been part of spiritual traditions, Indigenous communities, and ancestral cultures for generations. We still have much to learn from communities that uplift the connection between mind, body, and spirit, as well as the importance of prioritizing harmony and balance in our relationships and our interconnection to all things. We are grateful for the lessons of ancestors whose words came across many lineages to find their way into the practices we received in different social movement and healing circles, which we now share here. We honor these teachings and hope to be a small part of the work that forwards them along for the next seven generations.

We are so happy you have picked up this workbook, and we hope it becomes a living document in your life and/or organization and inspires collaborations that support and nourish your good work in the world!

PART I

PERSONAL WELL-BEING AND CONNECTION

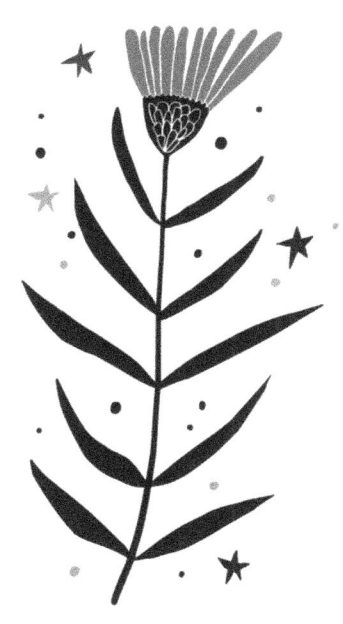

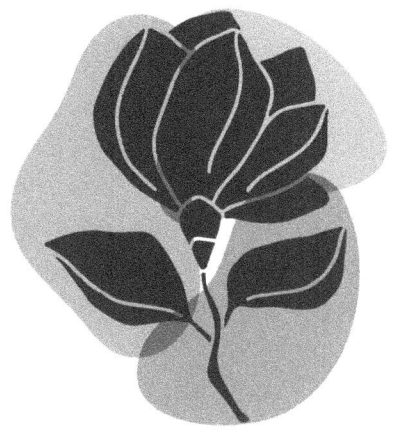

EMBODIED PRACTICES FOR SELF-REGULATION

As discussed in our accompanying anthology, *Practicing Liberation: Transformative Strategies for Collective Healing and Systems Change*, our bodies hold our stories. They carry the power and grace we acquire through our life experiences as well as the energy of unresolved trauma. Our body is our guidance system. It's like a GPS—when it's properly calibrated, it gives us accurate information about the outside world and how to move through it, when there's danger and we should retreat or fight, and when we're safe and we can settle. But when we are overburdened with trauma or stress, our body's signals can be unreliable and erratic. One word for this is *dysregulation*. This means that we are stuck in activation or shut down, or we go back and forth from one extreme to the other. When we are stuck in survival mode, overwhelm, or defense, our thinking (and feeling) is black and white. This can lead to conflict and poor communication. It's almost impossible to have nuance and see multiple sides to a situation when we're dysregulated, and it becomes very hard to relate to others and communicate effectively. When we can settle ourselves, we can gradually recalibrate our body's guidance system. We can collaborate, be accountable, communicate skillfully, thoughtfully connect, get creative, and be more effective in our work together.

In addition to connecting us to what is going on inside of us, embodied practices can help us manage the overwhelm that can come when we reconnect to our emotions. When we can feel settled in the face of intense emotions (both ours and those of other people), we are more likely to navigate the situation in a way that is better for everyone involved. Simple things like breathing, movement, and checking in with ourselves—individually or in groups—can help regulate the nervous system and thus change the energy of a meeting or one-on-one interactions. Understanding when we are triggered can allow us to take a moment to settle before we engage with someone; when we are settled, our communication will be more skillful. When everyone inside an organization understands that we are all carrying both hardships and strengths, and when we frontload curiosity and empathy for each other, we can find ways of being in the stress and chaos without turning on each other.

Embodied practices build up our capacity to be with discomfort without going into a trauma response. Trauma responses cause us to blame, shame, project, shut down, or lash out; they are never useful (unless you're in an actual life-threatening situation). Understanding how we respond to trauma is especially important when doing work around community suffering or social justice that exposes us to traumatic situations and circumstances. When we are not regulated in our body and mind, we can feel anxious, stressed, depressed, or just off. Our actions can be impulsive rather than deliberate, which often doesn't serve our best interest (or the interests of those around us). Self-regulation practices allow us to stay connected to each other amid great challenges, so we can be part of the solution.

Being self-regulated refers to being in a state of feeling grounded, centered, and present. It can also refer to feeling settled in ourselves. Self-regulation is not always a still or quiet state; we can be self-regulated while being active and engaged. We can dance, sing, and shake it off to regulate ourselves or we can practice quiet contemplation, meditation, or slow movement. The simple self-regulation practices in this workbook can support us in finding some peace in our body and mind amid stress or pressure. They can shift us out of dysregulation toward greater self-regulation and coherence inside ourselves. Practices like this can serve several purposes:

Care for self: Practicing ways to care for ourselves by soothing the nervous system and settling the body can mitigate burnout or exhaustion.

Effective communication: When we are regulated, we are more likely to relate to others in a skillful and authentic way that fosters trust and effective collaboration.

Accountability: When we can connect to what is going on inside of us, we are more aware of our motivations and actions.

Systems change: When we care for ourselves and each other, we have the strength and resilience to change oppressive systems (as opposed to settling into systems that are unjust).

The concept of self-care has been commodified by corporations and influencers trying to sell products and a superficial version of self-care that is often indulgent and affordable only to wealthy people. For frontline communities, self-care is, to borrow from Audre Lorde, an act of self-preservation. We see self-care as a form of actively supporting our own health and well-being, which is necessary if we want to be sustainable and effective in the long-haul work of collective social change. We also believe it is directly connected to community care and helps us show up fully and thoughtfully in the face of oppressive systems that don't support our well-being. We can't hope to magically build a world that takes care of its members better if we don't know how to take care of ourselves and each other, here and now, in practice for that world.

If you are experiencing stress, burnout, rage, grief, or disconnection, we encourage you to give yourself the permission to rest and tend to your individual well-being. We know it can feel difficult to find the time, space, and resources to engage in these practices, or to even acknowledge their worth against the backdrop of urgent community needs. However, personally practicing healing and care regularly helps build greater strength, resilience, and spaciousness so we can meaningfully connect with and take care of others.

These practices can be done regularly to build a strong foundation of centeredness and presence that can transform you over time; they can also be done on an as-needed basis in moments when you're feeling particularly stressed or overwhelmed. You do not need to do them in order, and you can choose to use just the ones that are most effective for you.

> *For some people, even simple practices like breathing or grounding can bring up a sense of overwhelm. This might be true for you if you are holding a lot of trauma in your body that you have not had space to feel. If you find any practices overwhelming, remember that you can stop at any time. Bringing your attention to something outside your body (see the following orienting practice), asking for support from a safe person, or seeking support from a qualified provider who understands trauma can help. The practices shared in this section are meant to help you be in your body in a way that isn't overwhelming, but they don't work for everyone right away. We all have different bodies and there's no one right way to find internal balance and regulation. We encourage readers to try different practices to find the one that best suits them.*

We suggest doing these as your own personal practice throughout your day and specifically in moments when you feel anxious, ungrounded, or uncentered. We also suggest incorporating them into group settings such as at the start of a meeting or work session. Consistently starting any group meeting with a short practice, even if it's just one breath, can shift the energy of the entire process; it can allow everyone to be a bit more present and connected. If you choose to do this collectively, you can take turns facilitating the exercises and reading the instructions so others can follow along. Remember to always make things like this optional so people feel like they have a choice as to whether to participate. All of the offerings here can be adapted based on the culture, conditions, time, space, and the needs of you and your group.

> **NOTE** *By encouraging settling we are not discouraging having big feelings. In fact, sometimes when we settle into ourselves, we realize we are angry or upset, and we can act or communicate from a place of being connected to what feels true for us in the moment with more skill. Being grounded while expressing our passionate feelings can allow us to communicate more effectively while still remaining flexible and open to other perspectives. These practices can be helpful when tension is high and people need a break to shift their energy. But, it's important not to use them as a subtle way to shame people who may be having big feelings or feeling frustrated. So be sensitive to when and how the practices are brought in.*

Orienting Practice —HALA KHOURI[1]

Orienting is about becoming present with the external environment. We need to have a certain amount of safety in our surroundings if we are going to settle our bodies. The following exercise is a visual orienting practice, but you can work with any of your senses (smell, hearing, touch, and even taste). Orienting to our external world can sometimes help us then orient to our internal world. Orienting outside of ourselves can also help pull us out of overwhelm if what's happening inside of us feels like too much; it can be a form of putting the brakes on or lowering the volume of intensity.

When orienting visually, make sure to slowly turn your head side to side and notice also what might be behind and above you. The movement of the head (slowly) can often feel settling. Also, don't orient to things you want to organize, clean up, or that you find unpleasant. Try to have an attitude of pure observation and curiosity instead.

Here are several ways to orient:

Orient to colors and textures: Simply notice the different colors and textures in the room.

Orient to a particular color: Look for four blue things in the room, then three brown things, then two yellow things, and one red thing.

Orient to objects: Notice and name the different objects you see in the room.

Orient to pleasant things: Find something that is pleasant to look at and really notice it.

Body Scan (Interoception)   —HALA KHOURI

The first step to any settling practice is realizing that we need it. *Interoception* is sensing what is happening inside of us. It can take practice to be good at interoception, but research shows that the better we are at knowing what's happening in our internal environment, the more skillfully and authentically we engage with our external environment.[2] Here are some simple ways to develop greater interoception.

Take a moment to check in with how your body is feeling. Start by noticing your sensations and breathing pattern. Notice if any emotions are present. You may feel nothing, and that is also information for you. It can be helpful to scan your body from the ground up. Start by noticing if you feel your feet and legs, your bum in the chair, and so on. Is your breath feeling shallow, deep, smooth, rough? Does anything feel tight or loose? We often tend to notice what feels bad or uncomfortable, so make sure you also look for what feels good or neutral. Notice if anything starts to settle or feel better simply by taking a moment to tune into yourself. You may also notice the opposite, that things emerge and get stronger because you are now noticing them. There's no wrong way to do this; just try to maintain an attitude of curiosity with yourself rather than judgment. Tuning into what is happening in your body will likely alert you to any self- or community-care practices you may want to invest in.

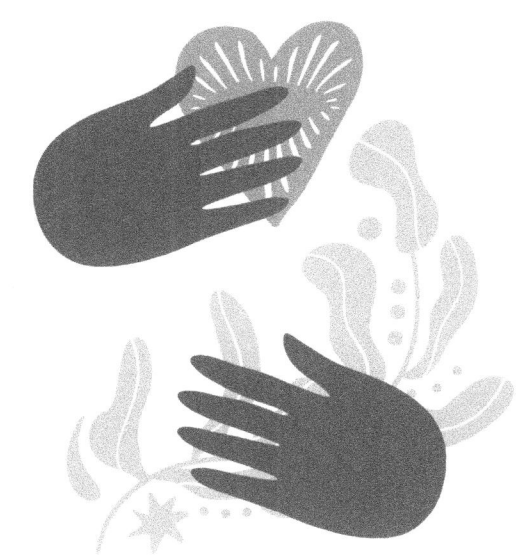

OPTIONAL

Place one hand on your heart and the other on your belly. Notice if anything settles when you do this. Take three, slow, deep breaths. Notice if anything settles further when you do this. Notice if the energy in the room changes after doing this with others.

DAILY INTEROCEPTION

Try to notice what is happening in your body throughout your day. You can use naturally occurring moments of pause (such as when stopping at a red light, waiting for your computer to load, waiting in line) or set an alarm to remind you a few times a day to pause and check in with your sensations.

Tapping   —HALA KHOURI

Many people find that tapping the body with the finger-tips, open palm, or loose fist helps settle or energize the body, both of which can be grounding. You can try this out yourself by finding a comfortable seated position in a chair or on the floor. With your fingers, gently tap the top of your head with both hands. Then move down to tapping your temples, then your forehead. Guide your fingers to now tap underneath your eyes, out to the jaw, and to the chin below your lip. Take both hands and tap the center of your chest, and then with loose fists, gently tap down the sides of your body, to your toes, and back up. Release your hands and notice your sensations. Does anything settle or become more spacious? How is your breathing? What else do you notice?

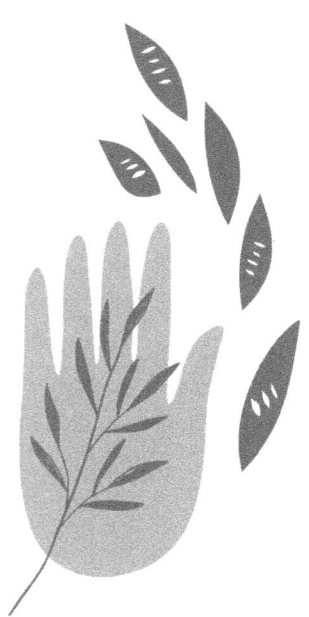

Shake It Out   —HALA KHOURI

This is a good one to do if you're feeling lethargic and need to move some energy or if you're feeling very amped up and need to release some energy so you can settle down. Bring your own intention to the movements!

Start by taking a few deep breaths. Then shake out your arms, shoulders, and elbows. Then your legs, knees, ankles, and thighs. You can shake out your hips and then bend and straighten your knees really fast to get a full body shake. You can bounce on your heels and pull energy up from the earth as you bounce and shake. You can make sounds and bounce around, anything that helps you shake things out. Do this for one or two minutes. When you finish, pause and feel your feet on the floor or your bum in your chair. Take a few very deep breaths allowing yourself to settle. Notice if you feel different now, and if so, how.

Seated Grounding Practice   —HALA KHOURI

Being grounded is about feeling supported and held. It can feel like you are connected to something solid and steady both outside of you and inside of you. Some people are naturally very grounded, and others tend to be a bit more floaty. When we are anxious or shut down, we often lose our sense of grounding. This practice can help you find it again.

Find a comfortable seated position. Bring your attention to the parts of your body that are touching the floor or chair. Notice these areas—perhaps your feet, the back of your thighs, your bottom, arms, or hands. If your feet are on the floor, gently press them down and notice how your legs feel. Are they strong? Weak? Heavy? Light? Feel your sitz bones on the chair or your back against the chair. Let yourself really be held. Allow your spine to lengthen the more you ground down, just like a tree that is able to rise to the sun as it deepens its roots. As you bring awareness to the places in your body that are being supported by the floor or chair, notice if anything settles in your body.

Standing Grounding Practice —HALA KHOURI

Stand with your feet a bit wider than hip-distance apart and your knees slightly bent. Start to sway side to side. Find a rhythm that feels good to you. Notice the shift in weight in your feet and how your legs feel. Tune in to your muscles and how they engage as you sway. Notice if anything settles in the rest of your body as you get more grounded.

Return to a still position. Take one hand and place it on your heart and the other on your stomach. Notice anything that feels settling, grounded, or kicks up your nervous system. Do not judge or try to fix but just notice. Take a few deep breaths. Let that breath circulate through your body.

Containment Practice —HALA KHOURI

Like a grounding practice, this one can also connect you to feeling held and supported. This is a good one to try when things feel overwhelming or out of control.

Cross your forearms in front of your body and squeeze your opposite arm with each hand. Gently squeeze your hands up the arms to your shoulders and back down the arms to your wrists. Notice if anything settles in your body or your breath deepens and if there is a particular part of the movement that feels especially good.

Mountain Pose Practice —BELOVED COMMUNITIES NETWORK

The mountain pose begins by facing your hips and shoulders forward, arms by your sides, palms facing your side body. Separate your feet, hip-distance apart, to distribute your weight to the balls of your feet. Gather energy from the earth, as if you are scooping it into the palms of your hands, and move your arms up slowly in front of your body with your palms facing inward, while breathing in through your mouth.

When you reach the height where your arms are stretched fully above your head, start gathering energy, this time from above, moving your arms in a downward motion in front of your body with your palms facing outward in the shape of a mountain, breathing out through the nose. Repeat these steps while facing your body to the left, then switch to turn toward your right, forming a mountain on each side.

Slow down the pace and do this a number of times in each direction. Remember to continue to breathe in through the mouth while moving energy up, and exhale through the nose while moving energy down. This may feel like an odd or reversed way of inhaling and exhaling, so try to stay centered as you practice this kind of intentional breathing; move the energy in multiple directions with the movement of your arms and the different directions you are facing.

Afterward, take a few minutes to reflect on this embodied practice and write down or share with another one to three words about how this practice might resonate with you, what you found challenging, and whether/how you felt the energy move while doing it.

Grounding Energy Healing Exercise —HAIZE HAWKE

1. Close your eyes and take a deep breath.
2. Focus your energy on the present moment.
3. Drop your shoulders.
4. Sit tall.
5. Put your fingertips together and hold them lightly together in a very comfortable position.

6. Then, breathe deeply.

7. Become the observer to your breath.

8. Scan your body for tightness or comfort and practice breathing to circulate air through your body.

It's okay to notice your thoughts—take a deep breath afterward to bring yourself into the moment to recognize that you can be whole, happy, and healthy in each individual moment. Breathe in peace. As you breathe out, breathe out tension, breathe out fear, breathe out small-mindedness, breathe out anything that doesn't serve you right now. For this exact moment, limit thinking and anger. Breathe in positivity and love. Breathe in more peace, breathe in light, and breathe out anxiety. Quiet your mind, letting go of thoughts.

Now as you breathe in, imagine that you're pulling all your scattered parts back home to yourself with your breath. Any energy that you left with another person, in another place, at another time—call it back in to yourself. Call it back in without thinking about it or trying; just feel your energy being drawn back to you. Bring what may have been left behind back from all those places and spaces. Every fractured piece is coming to fill you up and have you become whole with each breath. Feel your energy becoming more whole, more complete. Feel it becoming more coherent. See or feel it coming back together into wholeness, as if you were rewinding a movie or mending a pot that was broken—it's coming back. Release the things in the spaces that don't get you, that don't support you, that don't see you.

Taking a deep breath in, inhaling deeply, exhaling long, just breathe and continue seeing yourself as whole and complete—for just a little bit of time. When you are ready to feel your energy, your essence, begin to form a slight focus and put your attention at the midpoint of your chest, forehead, or anywhere else that feels natural.

Begin to form a slight focus at that point in your body. When it feels right, open your eyes and come back to this present moment in time. Feel the fingertips and the toes and then give your body just a gentle stretch and shake. Pause and absorb the benefits of your practice.

If there is something I would offer to anyone seeking to act on behalf of their own healing without benefit of external resources, it is practicing vagus nerve activation by breathing in to a count of four and breathing out to a count of six or more. This simple technique does not require formal meditation but has the capacity anywhere, anytime, to regulate the nervous system by way of breathing; it is an antidote to the fight/flight/freeze/appease response of a triggered sympathetic nervous system, to adrenal overload and fatigue, to overproduction of cortisol, and it balances the amygdala and hippocampus. I think of vagus breathing as a means of decolonizing our nervous systems through self-regulation of the trauma response, releasing stress, and activating the body's triune (heart-brain-gut) coherence, laying a foundation for anchoring from within that can impact how we stay present and grounded in the moment, respond to unpredictable circumstances, and hold agency by first establishing sovereignty of our own breath.

—VALORIE THOMAS[3]

Awakening the Kundalini   —HAIZE HAWKE

Hinduism teaches that each individual has *Kundalini*, a Sanskrit word for "coiled snake," that describes the spiritual energy that sits at the base of the spine. When the energy arises or awakens, the spiritual emergence can set greater intentions for individuals and the collective. Natural energy that stems unconsciously in the body can transform into positive energy that practitioners can utilize to set their intention. All of this stems from the diaphragm to the back of the spine, embodying all of the energy by changing our emotions. When we are actively breathing, we are activating the energy. A quick way to release this energy is to perform a technique called the *energetic Kundalini movement*.

Raise your hands in the air and rapidly bring them back down to your heart, repeating the movement as you speak aloud these words, with increasing energy:

YES! YES! YES! YES! I LOVE MYSELF!

YES! YES! YES! YES! I AM STRONG!

YES! YES! YES! YES! I AM POWERFUL!

YES! YES! YES! YES! I CLAIM MYSELF!

YES! YES! YES! YES! TO MY DREAMS!

YES! YES! YES! YES! TO MY PURPOSE!

YES! YES! YES! YES! YES! YES! TO ALL THAT IS FOR ME!

YES! YES! YES! YES! YES! YES! YES! YES!

Breathe. Feel the impact of your yeses. Receive this energy.

Mother-Earth Connection —HAIZE HAWKE

This exercise reflects our interdependent relationship to our environment and the earth. When you're still for a long period of time, your heartbeat can match the earth's heartbeat and your breathing, the way the earth breathes. If you've ever been some place high enough to see the trees, you see they are breathing; they're moving.

BREATHING WITH THE TREE

Sit at the base of a tree:

1. Lean your back against the tree.

2. Talk to the tree; speak whatever truth comes to you, from your heart, to the tree.

3. If you cannot find a tree, you can lie on the grass or the ground and focus on matching your breath and heartbeat to the center of the earth.

4. Place your whole body on the grass or even just put your hands on the grass. Feel the energy pass between you and the grass, or you and the tree.

5. Breathe for five minutes or more.

6. Try to match your heartbeat to the movement (in the tree, grass, earth).

7. When you are done, close your practice with gratitude for this moment of connection.

Walking Meditation on the Earth —SUSY ZEPEDA

When we walk like [we are rushing], we print anxiety and sorrow on the earth. We have to walk in a way that we only print peace and serenity on the earth . . . Be aware of the contact between your feet and the earth. Walk as if you are kissing the earth with your feet.

—THÍCH NHẤT HẠNH, *Peace Is Every Step*

Many of us always have a destination or a sense of purpose while walking. Sometimes that urgency and our need to get from point A to B makes us feel like we're operating as machines. How often do you take the time to feel the ground beneath your feet? Can you take a breath with each step? Do you ever pause to tap into the direction and intention of your footsteps? It can be difficult to consciously know the intention of where we're going when we are disconnected or in a rush, but taking a few minutes out of our day to pause and practice walking meditation can help us stay attentive while reconnecting our whole self back to the earth.

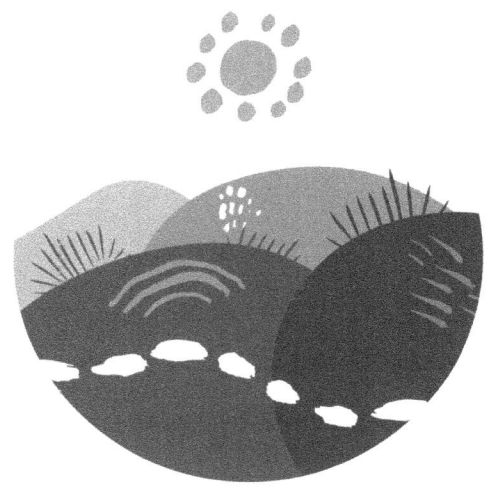

This practice can be done individually or as a group.

If you can, get on the grass, the sand, the dirt, or some form of the earth, and walk barefoot to feel the ground beneath your feet. Take your time to lift each foot from the ground and shift your weight from one foot to the other. Allow for the cleansing and rooting of your energy with that contact.

Give yourself time to breathe and pause. Breathe in, breathe out. It is okay to allow your mind to wander, yet be intentional about staying connected. If you encounter distractions, take a moment to notice these thoughts and feelings; then continue to bring your attention back to this walking meditation. Aim to focus on the sensations of being held by the earth, the clarity that arrives when we breathe deeply and consciously. Bring mindful awareness to walking, stillness, and gentle movements.

After you complete a simple, slow walk, you can reflect on this walking meditation with these questions:

1. What was the walking meditation like for you? How did it feel to slow down? Describe your experience.

2. What was it like walking with a sense of connectedness and intention?

3. What thoughts or sensations did you notice?

4. Did you have any distractions or feelings that came up for you during the walk? How did you redirect your energy to being present with the slow movement?

5. Can you get curious and learn from this practice about what may have challenged you?

_____

_____

_____

6. How might you bring the gentle wisdom of this practice into your day?

_____

_____

_____

PERSONAL REFLECTIONS

For many people, the desire to work on a specific social issue stems from personal experience with that issue. While taking action around that issue can be personally transformative and can even help to heal some wounds, sometimes unacknowledged trauma or unfinished healing can end up being unfairly projected onto others. *Radical healing* includes becoming more deeply aware of, caring for, and loving ourselves and others. As Thích Nhất Hạnh explains, "We should not try to help others in an effort to escape our own sorrow, despair, or inner conflict. If you are not peaceful and solid enough inside yourself, your contributions will not be as useful. We must first practice mindfulness and grow compassion in ourselves, so that peace and harmony are in us, before we can work effectively for social change."[4] In other words, if we seek to aid in the liberation of others, we must also commit to the ongoing work of internal liberation and caring for ourselves.

This section is an invitation to deepen your own awareness and personal self by reflecting on how your individual body and nervous system function. Some of the previous embodied practices may reveal to you things about your own mind-body connection that you weren't fully aware of. For example, you may find that some practices activate you rather than settle you; or that you didn't even realize that you weren't grounded when you checked in with yourself. You may also discover new layers of awareness around your own physiological and psychological tendencies and what helps you to become self-regulated.

Self-reflection is a powerful tool that lays the groundwork for internal awareness, accountability, effective communication, and collaboration. Understanding your own GPS is important in navigating how you show up for yourself, others, and the work you are engaging in. If you tried some of the practices in the previous section, reflect on some of these questions:

1. Which practices did you find most effective in supporting you to settle and regulate?

2. Do other practices that you are already familiar with work well for you?

3. How do these practices support you?

4. How might using these practices support how you show up for others and the work you engage in?

5. When can you incorporate these practices into your workday?

6. Are there group settings where these practices might be useful to do together?

Body Map   —HALA KHOURI

Draw an outline of your body; you can do this on regular-sized paper, or you can get life-sized paper and get someone to actually trace your body. This doesn't have to be perfect or realistic.

1. Using different colors, color in and add words, images, and/or designs to the various parts of your body.

2. Here are some possible questions to inspire your process:

    a. What does this part of my body hold?

    b. What does this part of my body remember?

    c. What does this part of my body need?

    d. How does this part of my body feel?

    e. If this part of my body could speak, what would it say?

3. There's no wrong way to do this! Track your own body as you do this, and see what emerges.

4. When you finish, look at the overall image and notice what it teaches you about yourself. Consider what you can do to take care of your body's needs.

MY BODY MAP

Stress-Goal Curve —HALA KHOURI

When we are overburdened by stress, we may find that embodied practices and meditation aren't as effective as we need them to be. They can feel like trying to put out a fire with teaspoons of water. When we get to this place, which often looks like exhaustion, illness, or relationship breakdown, we may need to take a step back and make some significant changes. This might mean taking time off, getting more support, reassessing strategy and mission on an organizational level, and so on.

The following adapted graph maps what is typically called the *stress-performance curve*.[5] This aims to decipher where you are in terms of your optimal stress zone—that is, the sweet spot in your life in which there is the right amount of stress to mobilize your goals but not too much so that you feel frazzled or burnt out (or on the flip side, too little stress/challenge so that you feel bored or apathetic). It is important to moderate stress because having too much or too little of it is not good for us. We each have our own unique optimal zone in which we are navigating enough challenge to feel inspired, effective, and on purpose. You can also think of this as your "zone of resilience," where life feels manageable and you feel balanced.

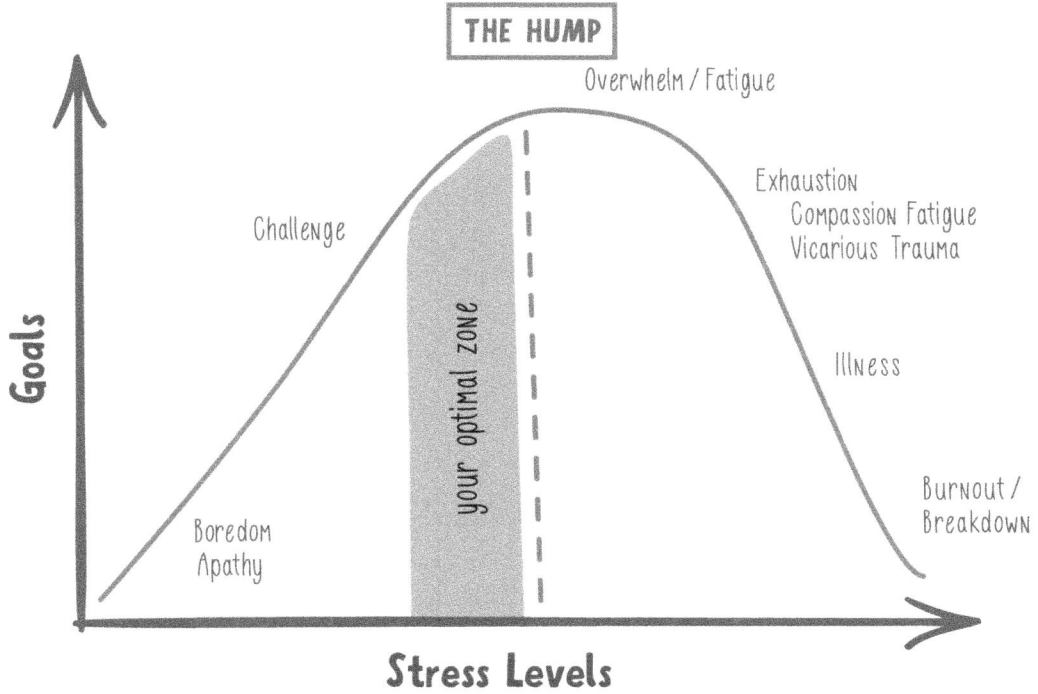

When the stress load gets too high, it has a deleterious impact on our work, well-being, and relationships. Many things that take us outside our optimal zone can be external and not in our control; it's important to acknowledge this and not blame ourselves for our burnout or overwhelm. Simultaneously, we *can* get curious about what we can control, and how we might cope with high levels of stress, both by working to change the circumstances causing the stress where we can and by addressing our own internal habits and tendencies, which can contribute to our overwhelm.

Using this graph, reflect on your current goals and stress levels. Consider "goals" in a personal and nuanced way that reflects your values and what you want to move toward. We don't want to assume that productivity is the goal for everyone. That assumption can be deeply problematic when people's worth is measured only in their productivity without questioning its cost; this assumption also fails to recognize other goals people may be aspiring to in their work. You might consider goals such as acting with greater integrity, engaging in skillful action and words, and finding flow in your work process or relationships. Feel free to fill in your own words for what your goals are (on the vertical axis) and then assess what degree of stress you experience pertaining to achieving these goals.

After mapping yourself on this graph, what information does this reflection offer you?

1. Where on the curve are you currently?

2. How do you know if/when you are outside of your optimal zone?

    Behaviors:

    Emotions:

    Thoughts:

    Physical symptoms:

    Relationships:

3. If you are out of your zone, what can you commit to right now to help you get back into it?

_____

_____

_____

4. How is your experience of yourself, others, or work altered when you are in your optimal zone?

_____

_____

_____

5. What are you already doing that supports you to manage your stress?

_____

_____

_____

Critical Reflection on Radical Healing of Self and Community — TESSA HICKS PETERSON

Extractive and oppressive culture norms can lead changemakers to struggle with prioritizing care for ourselves. Sometimes we cannot meet our basic needs due to unjust circumstances that are outside of our control, and it is important to identify when that is the case. Other times, self-care is accessible, but not prioritized, which means we must intentionally make time and space to foster such care. Avoiding self-judgment, reflect on each of the following foundational domains of personal well-being and consider which ones you are prioritizing and which ones you may want to focus on more.

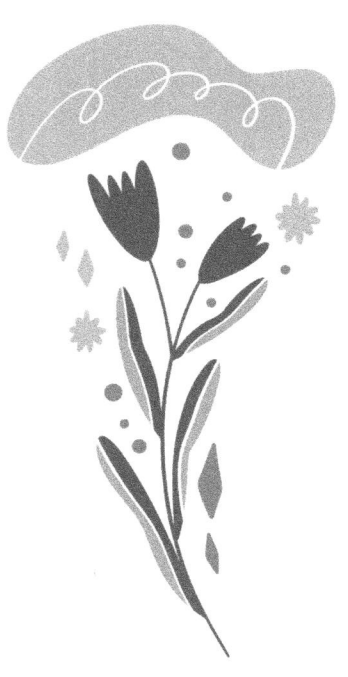

Safety: To support your body, mind, and heart to feel safe, cultivate and spend time in relationships and surroundings that allow you to settle into yourself and feel secure—physically, emotionally, mentally, and spiritually.

Nourishment: Support your physical body by eating foods that nourish you whenever available. Allow meals to be a source of connection by eating with people you love, without haste, or by eating in solitude with mindfulness in gratitude. Remember to stay hydrated and drink plenty of water each day.

Sleep: Protect your sleep as best you can and foster good sleep hygiene by unplugging from devices at least thirty minutes before bed and using relaxation techniques such as meditation or visualization to prepare your body for quality slumber. Getting adequate quality sleep is vital to our well-being.

Exercise: Move your body every day! If your lifestyle doesn't naturally include physical movement, try to set aside at least thirty minutes to walk, dance, or exercise in whatever way feels good to you.

Also consider:

Media Hygiene: Constant media consumption can be detrimental to well-being by keeping us in overwhelm and hypervigilance. A best practice is to turn off all unnecessary alerts and take in news at designated times of your day, not throughout your whole day. Limit social media usage, unplug from devices whenever possible, and curate your social media intentionally.

Healing and Reflective Practices: Incorporate practices that cultivate healing and reflection in your life. This can include individual things like journaling, therapy, bodywork, spending time in nature, contemplative practices like prayer and meditation, and other healing modalities. This also includes practices done with others that help us feel connected and supported.

Creative Practices: Being creative and playful is a powerful way to strengthen our well-being and imagine new futures. Simple things like making art, listening to music, dancing, cooking, and even just playing can be revitalizing and offer spaces for community connection and meaning making.

Community-Care Practices: Rev. Jen Bailey says, "social change moves at the speed of relationships and relationships move at the speed of trust." Participating in practices that build trusting relationships and that provide the opportunity and power of offering care and receiving care from others can greatly enhance individual and collective well-being.

What comes up for you while you are reading this list? Answer some of the following questions to make space for both your critical reflections and your hopes for yourself related to this topic.

1. Which of these self-care practices or community-care practices do you engage in regularly? If you resist such practices, why might that be? Can you become curious about this resistance?

2. What else could you add to this list to adapt it to your personal needs and desires?

3. What practices help you to be present, vulnerable, and listen well in the midst of more challenging community change work?

4. How can you support movements or communities that you are a part of to integrate self- and community-care values and practices?

_____

_____

_____

What Does Self-Care Mean to You? — HALA KHOURI

Sometimes our unconscious beliefs about self-care can keep us from doing the things we know would support us. Reflect on these questions for yourself.

1. What did you learn about self-care in your family of origin? (What was modeled to you or what were you explicitly told about it?)

_____

_____

_____

2. How do these beliefs help or hinder you in your life today?

_____

_____

_____

3. What belief about self-care would you like to embrace? Write something that is bold and inspiring even if you don't fully believe it yet.

4. Do you already do things that make you feel good, grounded, or more present (even if you don't call them self-care practices)?

5. How can you connect self-care to community-care practices? (Hint: Find a friend or colleague to do some of the practices with or to have as an accountability partner.)

Draw a picture to express what your life could look and feel like if you embraced an affirming attitude toward self-care. Remember that this includes getting support from (and giving support to) your community. We are all part of a web of mutuality and care! Your picture can be abstract or literal, and it can include words if you like. You may even choose to create a collage to explore and express your ideas!

MY OPTIMAL SELF-CARE

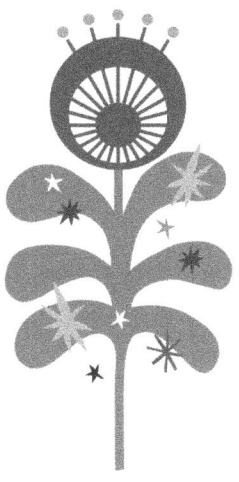

MEDITATION AND CONTEMPLATIVE PRACTICES

Meditation, mindfulness, and contemplative practices have their roots in many cultures and spiritual traditions. Various traditions have different goals for meditation ranging from cultivating present moment awareness to union with the sacred, from expanding consciousness to opening hearts. Having breath and body awareness and bringing this mindful awareness to the present moment are central to most meditation practice. For many, meditation and contemplative practices bring about a greater sense of grounding, presence, and awareness that can help increase attention, attunement, and connection in different ways.

Although they sound simple, these practices may be challenging as we usually find ourselves reacting to every noise we hear and itch we feel. The aim, however, is to make space for whatever arises, without judgment. When distracting thoughts arise, you can imagine them floating by like a cloud; you can notice the impermanent nature of them, rather than grasping at them as if they are a concrete and fixed experience. Though these practices are about staying present and bringing our awareness to whatever arises, it's really knowing that the mind has wandered *and* coming back to the present moment that is the practice of meditation. Whether we are able to notice our awareness wandering and bring it back to the present moment one hundred times or one time in our meditation practice, it's all good medicine!

You can use any of the somatic practices from the "Embodied Practices" section of the book to prepare for meditation. You may choose to engage in this section's initial meditation practices to make yourself aware of your breath and body, also known as your *anchor*, or, like the subsequent practices in this section suggest, to help yourself focus and cultivate awareness of and presence to a specific topic. Find the ones that resonate for different moments in time. You may choose to practice this in a private way or in a group with others, known as a *sangha*, in order to build a community around a shared practice.

This section contains meditations and reflections shared with us by various meditation teachers on different themes, drawing on specific practices from the Theravada Buddhist tradition, including the heart practices of the Brahmaviharas.

Preparing Your Body for Meditation Practice   —LESLIE BOOKER

Students of meditation are often instructed to "find a comfortable position, and close your eyes." The problem with this instruction is that many of us have no idea what "comfortable" feels like in our body or our nervous system. This is not a personal failing; rather, it follows a narrative that meditation practice is supposed to be uncomfortable, and therefore difficult. What follows are some foundational instructions to support us having ease and comfort in a formal meditation practice. There are instructions on how to find ease in the four classic postures of meditation, and how to find our anchor in each. The anchor is a very important part of our practice, because it gives us a place to go back to when we've noticed the mind has wandered.

THE FOUR POSTURES

A formal meditation practice has four classic postures: sitting, standing, walking, or lying down. These are a direct instruction in the Satipatthana Sutta, the foundational discourse in the Theravada Buddhist tradition. At the time of this writing, in the Insight/Western Theravada lineage, some of us are moving away from terms like *sitting* or *walking meditation*, knowing that not everyone has access to these forms. We are starting to use words like *still practice* and *moving practice*. I will be using both these terms to accommodate as many bodies as I am able in this offering.

Lying Down | Still Practice

This is a posture that is not typically offered on meditation retreats because of its great potential for allowing the practitioner to fall asleep! Lying down is a great posture for you if you are recovering from insult or injury, or if you feel like you're carrying the weight of the world on your shoulders. This posture allows for the earth to bear witness, to hold whatever you are not able to. This is not meant to be practiced if you are sleepy.

How to Practice

Lie down, typically on your back; lying on your side is also okay.

I like to bend my knees and plant the bottoms of my feet into the earth, typically a bit wider than my hips. This allows for the base of my spine to rest firmly on the ground, protecting my lower back.

Slightly tuck your chin down toward your heart so that the crown on your head lifts up and the spine elongates.

Rest your arms and hands on your belly, the heart, down by your side, or out to the side, whichever is most comfortable for you. Some find it useful to root the back of the upper arms to the ground with fingertips pointing up toward the ceiling, which can be very helpful in keeping us awake during this practice.

Eyes can be open, holding a soft focus, looking down toward your belly or tip of the nose, or closed altogether.

Anchor

In this posture, the anchor can be the bottoms of your feet, your back body (movement of lungs, lower back, etc.), or the back of the head as you rest on the ground. This is also a great posture for watching the belly rise and fall as your breath moves through.

After you've completed your practice, bring your knees toward your chest and roll to one side of your body, with your bottom arm extended so that your head can rest on it.

Place the opposite hand on the floor in front of your heart, and when you're ready, press into this hand to support yourself in coming to an upright posture.

Sitting | Still Practice

This is the typical posture you'll see folks put their body into when it's time to meditate. There is no particular added value to this posture; it's just the one that we see on magazine covers! It is a useful posture if your body is feeling upright and able and so you can feel a connection to the ground beneath you.

How to Practice

If you sit on the ground, the sitz bones (the bones we feel when we're sitting on our bottom) should be a bit higher than the knees so that the natural curvature of the spine is slightly exaggerated. Sitting on the edge of a meditation cushion, or on a folded blanket or two, should be enough to allow the lumbar spine (the lower back) to curve so that the belly can be soft and kind of fall forward. You can also sit on a chair or a bed.

From this foundation, the body is being held up by your skeleton, not your muscles. Your legs can be crossed so that your ankles are placed one in front of the other, not crisscross applesauce or in Lotus (with the ankles resting on top of the legs).

If your knees are not connecting to the earth, put a bit more cushion under your bottom instead of under the knees. After you're complete with your practice, you might find it useful to stretch your legs out for a moment before you stand up.

The hands are typically resting palms down on top of the upper legs, but your hands can also be resting on your heart, or palm inside of palm with thumbs touching. Eyes can be open holding a soft focus, looking down toward your belly or tip of your nose, or closed altogether.

Anchor

Your anchor in this posture could be the weightedness of your bottom resting on the earth, or the hands resting on your lap. If you find it more beneficial to anchor outside of the body, you can use sense doors like sound, smell, or touch. For example, you could use touch to feel the nubbiness of a blanket between your fingers or the texture of socks around your feet.

Standing | Still Practice

This is a great practice if your body is feeling sleepy and could use a bit more energy. Some folks might start in a sitting posture, and then stand up halfway through their practice because of discomfort or because they find themselves falling asleep. This can be used as a respite from the sitting | still practice or as its own posture.

How to Practice

Stand up and have your feet a bit wider than your hips. This is specific to each body; play around with the width of your feet and see what offers the most stability.

Your knees should be softly bent so they're not locked into place.

Your arms can be down by your side, hand on heart, or clasped in front of you or behind your back.

You might notice that it's a bit challenging to keep your balance with your eyes closed; if that's the case, hold your eyes open with a soft focus, or look down to a spot on the ground.

Anchor

Your anchor in this posture could be touching to the floor the four corners of the bottom of your feet or the weightedness of your pelvic bone.

Walking | Moving Practice

This is a great practice to use if your body has a lot of energy that needs to be moved through, and it also provides a great balance if you have been doing a lot of still practice. Walking or moving practice is a physical experience that can complement our still practice. This can be incredibly useful for moving things through that might have gotten stuck in stillness. This practice can manifest as a walking meditation practice, yoga, qi gong, tai chi, or any other mindful movement practice. It's also been found that folks with limited or less mobility can light up the same part of the brain that happens with movement with the *intention* to move. You can also move your fingers, hands, or arms, rather than your legs and feet. The instruction I offer is for a classic walking meditation practice.

How to Practice

Begin with the instructions from standing meditation practice.

Typically the instruction for a walking practice is to walk no more than about ten to twenty steps before pausing and then slowly turning around to walk back in the direction you came from.

Some might say to themselves as they move their feet, "lifting, moving, placing" to keep their minds focused on their practice.

The intention here is to kind of bore the mind so that it becomes more collected. If we're going for a walk without this intention, the mind will get distracted with all the new things and experiences it will encounter on its journey.

Sometimes folks will begin to walk very slowly, paying attention to the nuance and mechanics of walking. This can be of interest to some folks and can be quite agitating to others.

For others, walking fast, even a running practice, might be a better fit to excise some of the energy. Here, saying to yourself "placing, placing, placing" as the feet hit the ground might be useful to keep the mind collected.

Some folks might continue to move quickly or eventually slow down.

The pace doesn't matter as long as there is mindfulness present.

Please do keep your eyes open, and move your arms to support your natural walk.

Anchor

The anchor in this practice could be connecting your feet to the earth or the breath as you find rhythm and cadence in your movement.

Preparing Your Nervous System for Meditation Practice
—LESLIE BOOKER

Now that you have found the posture that brings some ease to the body, it's time to bring your awareness to your nervous system, which is the part of our body that alerts us to danger, safety, arousal, and settling. For some reason, this is typically left out in meditation instruction, but it is integral to making sure that all the parts of us are ready to drop into meditation practice. Over the years, I've found myself borrowing resourcing or orienting practices from Somatic Experiencing[6] to integrate into my meditation practice, which are similar to the initial activities provided in this workbook's "Embodied Practices for Self-Regulation."

HOW TO PRACTICE

After choosing one of the four meditation postures that works best for your body (and this can change from day to day), take some time to notice how you feel in your body beyond just how your muscles and joints feel. Notice if your belly is rising and falling, the expansion and contraction of your chest, if there is a tightness or stickiness. Developing an intimacy with the overall quality of your breath and body is a great way to set yourself up for your meditation practice. Continue to notice your sensations in all the parts of your body and where you feel settled, activated, numb, or solid. What other words would you use to describe the felt sense of your body, the physical sensations of your body in this present moment?

1. Keeping your eyes open, begin to slowly turn your head from right to left, and vice versa.

   As you do, notice the different colors you are seeing: the shadow, light, warmth, and coolness of colors.

2. Notice the natural elements: the light coming through a window, the rain, the wind blowing through trees. The folks that might be moving through your homes, a pet, houseplants.

   You can slowly turn your head, chin hovering over shoulders, for several minutes as you observe these things.

3. When you feel complete, pause.

   Turn your head upward to notice the space above you.

   Turn your head to the right and to the left to notice the space on either side of you.

   Notice the depth of your space: what is in front of you and what is behind you.

4. When you feel complete again, you can rest your eyes (keeping them open in a soft focus, looking down to a spot on the ground, or closing them completely) to begin your formal meditation practice.

The formal meditation practice, in whatever posture is used, involves bringing awareness to the present moment. This can be enhanced by softening and expanding the breath and attempting to clear the mind of its habit of grasping onto thoughts (regrets about the past or worries about the future) in order to become more fully present and aware of the moment.

Mudita for the Movement   —JACOBY BALLARD

Mudita, the practice of sympathetic joy, is a Buddhist practice, part of the four Brahmaviharas that also include loving kindness, compassion, and equanimity. Mudita is to be completely here and present for the delights, celebrations, pleasures, and successes, while not being attached to their longevity or permanence. Everything we love at some point will be lost. Mudita is a practice of really living in the present moment—to notice the goodness, brilliance, beauty of right now. It's all around us. It's the slanted light at dusk. It's yet another person waking up to the history and prevalence of white supremacy in our world. It's the fabulous gay-looking mimosa flower that delights me each July. It's the passion of an artist flowing in their craft.

It is so important to celebrate our wins. It increases our resilience as individuals, and as organizations, institutions, and communities. Joy is not an indulgence in service or social justice work; it is essential. How do you practice joy?

Our sacred task is to pause, to let moments of joy sweep us off our feet, to deepen our breath and pay attention. Our nervous systems are wired with a negativity bias, and we can really see it in change work; we are so good at critique, at noticing the holes, at sharp analysis. But what are our practices when a patient near death survives? When a beloved teenager turns a corner out of anxiety into a self-regulated state? When we do indeed save a sacred parcel of land from an oil pipeline? What do we do, collectively and individually, when a terrible bill is not passed by our state's house of representatives?

Even though our human nervous systems (and, thus, human-designed organizations) have this negativity bias, neuroplasticity demonstrates that we can always rewire—what we practice grows stronger. The more we celebrate and practice presence with the good stuff— the campaign wins, the inherent goodness of our neighbors—the better we get at noticing it. The more we notice it, the lighter we feel, because we are aware of the ten thousand joys, and not just the ten thousand sorrows.[7] This enhances our resilience, and we are able to do our nursing, social work, social change work, and healing work from a place of love and commitment, which is ultimately a more sustainable guide than grief and rage. Grief and rage are important, and we must not neglect these potent emotional states. We just cannot live there, individually or collectively.

What's more is that the practice of mudita invites you to take in the joy of others—the publishing of a paper by a colleague in another field, the success of an organization in another movement, the seating of another brilliant woman of color into US Congress—whether or not you yourself had anything to do with it. This joy is not just "their" joy; it is the joy of humanity, and you are invited to celebrate!

Now the crux of this practice is to not get attached. There will be a political backlash at some point. Your candidate will be voted out of office. An incredible leader will suffer hardship, be shamed or blamed, or even die. This is inevitable; this is the law of impermanence that invites us to seize this precious moment to celebrate and take in this pleasure! Don't miss it!

Become aware of the joys, delights, and pleasures that have touched your life recently. Remind yourself that you are so deserving of joy, just like every other being on the planet. Let your joy be sensual—sense the taste, the texture, the sound, the look, the smell of it.

MUDITA MEDITATION

Find a meditation posture that suits you—sitting in a chair or upon a cushion, lying down, or even standing. Holding your joys in your awareness, offer the following phrase:

May I be present to and fully take in my joy.
May I remember that this is just for now, not forever.
May I be fully here for my own pleasure and success.

Now consider someone whom it is relatively easy for you to rejoice with and actively recognize whatever joy or success is present in their lives. Imagine that person in your mind's eye and begin to silently offer this person the same phrase:

May I be present to and fully take in your joy.
May we both remember that this is just for now, and not forever.
May I be fully here for your pleasure and success.

Continue to offer these words for several minutes, and then return your attention to your heart, to check in and notice what has arisen. Following this, begin to offer mudita to a neutral person (someone you feel neither warmth nor coldness toward)—perhaps a colleague whom you haven't yet connected with deeply. Next, offer mudita to a difficult person, someone with whom you have active conflict. Finally, offer mudita to someone you might feel jealous or envious of.

Over time this practice diminishes the tendencies of the mind toward comparison, jealousy, and judgment; it enhances our resilience and allows us to be motivated by commitment and joy. Joy is a human need.

Forgiveness in Fellowship   —JACOBY BALLARD

It has been said that "forgiveness means giving up all hope of a better past."[8] Forgiveness is lightening our load, letting go of the burden of wishing something hadn't happened. World events or national events may impact us greatly and leave us exhausted and under-resourced, such as the five-hundred-plus anti-queer, anti-trans bills proposed in the US state legislatures in 2023, or the racial justice reckoning of 2020 brought about by the murder of George Floyd. Forgiveness is an important practice in medical settings, social service settings, and social justice organizations because difficult events occur and conflicts inevitably arise in relationships with colleagues, coworkers, employees, and bosses. We might have different ideas of strategy, or hold different identities so that the same event affects each of us quite differently. If we aren't mindful and attentive of our thoughts, words, and actions, we may hurt each other, and, of course, our capacity for mindfulness is greatly reduced when we are under stress.

In social justice work and helping professions, often there is a beautiful, profound, unattainable aspiration toward harmlessness. It guides our work to imagine a new way, to not create avoidable suffering, to not replicate harmful systems, to intervene rather than be a bystander. At the same time, we can set for ourselves unattainably high standards, and then we fail ourselves and one another. Sometimes we break apart silently, and sometimes people committed to doing really good work are called out and publicly humiliated. Surprisingly, this is sometimes easier than reckoning with our inherent imperfection and the inevitability of mistakes, even in the movements and institutions in which we seek refuge and healing. Rather than seeing these moments as breaks, obstacles, or misfortune, we might shift to see these as opportunities to slow down, learn, and heal. Forgiveness creates an essential time of self-reflection and internal accountability, which then enables and fosters the lasting change that we seek because we are vulnerably and transparently learning from our own mistakes and those of others, transforming ourselves and our world rather than resting in a place of judgment.

Pain is an unavoidable part of life, and forgiveness lights a way forward toward healing. Forgiveness invites us to consider the context of someone's life, that they too are a student, so that we learn ways of wisdom and freedom in a complicated and unhealthy world while also not neglecting our own feelings. Forgiveness removes the illusion that we could exist in this world and not participate in systems of oppression, or not cause harm—we too are implicated and imperfect—and forgiveness grants us permission to be human in this way.

In approaching forgiveness, I invite you to consider the great mistakes of your life, the ways you have betrayed or dishonored yourself, and also the flawed patterns that lead to suffering in our society. Consider forgiveness to be an investment in our creativity—if we go, deeply and courageously, into the mistakes and pain rather than avoiding, denying, judging, dismissing, we release our resistance and enter a tender space of imagination and vision. We need our greatest imagination and vision; and so as we free ourselves of the burden of how things should have been, we invoke our greatest gift and magic.

FORGIVENESS MEDITATION

Make sure you are in a meditation posture that works for you where you are able to be present and open. Begin to feel into your heart center with curiosity. Consider what you are up for, if you can turn toward profound suffering or only the small stuff on a day like today. When you are ready, begin offering forgiveness in the following directions, allowing time at the end to sit quietly with what arose.

Offering forgiveness toward yourself:

For any way that I have caused harm to myself,
I forgive myself.
May I allow myself to be a student of life and to make mistakes.
May I forgive myself,
And if I cannot do so in this moment,
May I be able to forgive myself in the future.

Asking for forgiveness from those you've harmed:

For any way that I have caused harm to you,
I ask for your forgiveness.
May you accept me with my imperfections and mistakes.
May you allow me to learn from my actions.
I ask for your forgiveness,
And if you cannot forgive me in this moment,
May you be able to forgive me in the future.

Offering forgiveness to those who have harmed you:

For any way that you have caused harm to me,
Knowingly or unknowingly,
In thought, word, or deed,
I forgive you.
May I allow you, too, to be a student of life and to make mistakes.
May I recognize your humanity, in the midst of my pain.
May my forgiveness soften any difficulties between us.
May I forgive you,
And if I cannot do so in this moment,
May I be able to forgive you in the future.

Directing forgiveness toward a greater suffering (destruction, tragedy, violence, abuse, war):

For any way that I have been unable to be present with,
And respond skillfully to,
The pain and suffering of our world,
My own pain, and that of others,
May I hold the pain with compassion,
And offer forgiveness for the way things are, and the way things have been.

There are layers and layers to forgiveness, but it doesn't mean that you're condoning the harm that you and your community experienced. Notice any type of resistance that you experience from the discomfort of forgiveness. It is okay to recognize if you are unable to forgive someone or something during this moment of time. It is okay to allow whatever feelings arise that are associated with this practice around forgiveness. Continue to breathe into your awareness of what is arising and how this process has felt.[9]

CRITICAL REFLECTION QUESTIONS

1. How can you encourage your heart to offer forgiveness toward someone or something for causing harm?

2. How does this practice of forgiveness feel in your body?

_____

_____

_____

3. How did you feel during and after the meditation?

_____

_____

_____

4. What is present in your heart?

_____

_____

_____

Equanimity for Equity   —JACOBY BALLARD

Equanimity is a practice I have struggled with and yet I believe it resources us, keeps our aspirations in check, invites us to let go rather than hold on tight. The boundary to our freedom is what we can make peace with or not. Fighting our history, what has led to this moment, wishing it were different—the slavery, genocide, millennia of control of women's bodies, the abuse within families or spiritual lineages—does not make it go away, does not dissipate it, does not heal it. Equanimity allows us to set down the fight, to accept that this current reality, these particular circumstances, these relationships, is what we have inherited; it is not any other way. Thinking and rethinking the past does not change it. We can learn from the past, certainly, and we must. Equanimity involves a peaceful perspective from the horizon, with a grand view, from a mountain top, or it involves considering the course of five hundred years of humanity, not just the four or eight years of a country.

Equanimity also encourages curiosity and a sense of awe: How did we get here, and what the heck could happen next? Wow!

I offer this practice here in this workbook because so much of social change work is framed as "the struggle," the fight, a campaign as a battle. We are fighting reality, and I wonder if that is the best way forward. What if we yielded, as one does in aikido? What if we wove a web with the intact, healthy strands that we've received from history rather than building a wall? What is possible if we set down the fight, the reactivity, the "this can't be happening!" and admit that this indeed is what is happening, and what is the most skillful way forward, out of harm and toward liberation?

Equanimity does not just pertain to the systems that we want to change. It is also relevant and useful in our relationships within institutions, organizations, and businesses; it is encouraging us to accept one another for who we are and what we are becoming, and to see the full picture of one another's humanity, removing pedestals. Someone in the seat next to you may have just woken up to the entrenched reality of police violence. Your neighbor's kid may have just come out as trans. Your beloved's sister may have just lost her wife suddenly. A city may have just passed a resolution to care deeply for its unhoused citizens. The US Supreme Court may have just passed a landmark ruling on immigration. Equanimity invites us to be present in this moment, and it also invites us to not map anything from this moment onto the next. As Buddhist teacher Sylvia Boorstein offers (quoting Buddhist teacher Gil Fronsdal), "This is what's happening now. Let's see what happens next."[10]

Lastly, equanimity invites us to let go of any illusion of "making someone happy" or to imagine that we can make anyone feel any kind of way. Their emotions and their liberation are their business. We can hold space, offer compassion, answer a call when it comes, but someone else's open heart, wisdom, and skillful words and actions are up to them. In this aspect of equanimity, we admit that there is only one thing we have power over, and that is ourselves. We can't make anyone feel better, or wake up, or have joy in their lives. There is such freedom in this! We are responsible for ourselves, and we are in a net of interdependence and responsible for our corner of it, but we cannot do the internal or external work for someone else.

Does equanimity sound relevant to what you are working on in the hospital, the social work arena, your organization or business? What possibility could it unlock? As with all practices, you are invited to not just take my word for it, but to try it on, see what works, keep what does, and leave the rest. Let's practice.

EQUANIMITY MEDITATION

Find your way into a preferred meditation posture. Breathe some deep breaths, sighing out through the mouth. Invite yourself to feel into your experience with whatever has rocked your boat recently as you continue breathing deeply.

Next, begin to offer these phrases to yourself, repeating them again and again for a set period of time, perhaps five to ten minutes:

This is what is happening.
May I learn to be with reality as it is, rather than how I might like it to be.
May I remain steady among the comings and goings of life.

Next direct your attention toward what is going on for people around you.

Equanimity isn't passivity but rather a warm acceptance of the way things are. In offering equanimity out in different directions, we remind ourselves that each person is in charge of their own liberation; despite our care, waking up, finding happiness or well-being is up to them.

Offer the following phrases to people in the categories of benefactor, neutral person, loved one, and difficult person, considering what may be rocking their lives. Work with each category of person for a set number of minutes, setting a timer for yourself if you like.

I care for you, but I cannot stop you from suffering.
May I hold your joys and sorrows with equanimity.
All beings are responsible for their own happiness.
May I remain rooted in the wind.

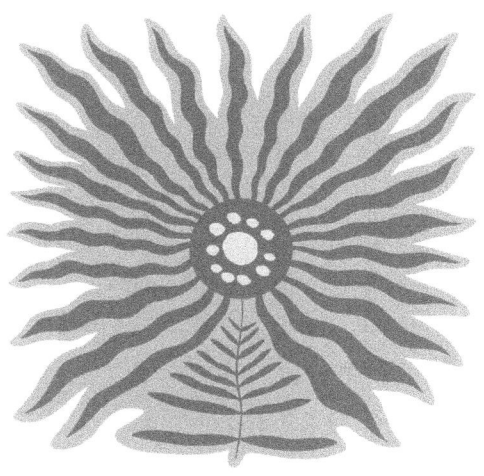

CRITICAL SELF-AWARENESS

Critical self-awareness is how we understand and know ourselves beyond our own personal mind, body, and spirit. It's an invitation to expand our sense of self so that we can see that we are all part of a larger social and cultural context that shapes us. Paulo Freire coined the term *conscientization*, or critical consciousness, to refer to the awareness of the sociopolitical context that shapes us.[11] A healing justice paradigm asks us to consider what has impacted us on a personal, interpersonal, and systemic level and how that influences our actions, perceptions, and relationships. It also invites us to structure our organizations around norms and practices that allow us to work together in ways that don't replicate harmful dynamics so our work together can be innovative, effective, and transformative.[12]

This process includes noticing the shape of our lives, including where systems of power are used against rather than with or for us; where structures limit our flourishing, access, and equitable experience; and where we have ingested such conditioning into our own thoughts and behaviors.[13] Here we get into the nitty-gritty of the values and culture, day-to-day assumptions, and community standards that we abide by that do not in fact serve our desired purposes. We can join others engaging in this change work to do this inventory at the personal level—including how we are personally situated in sociopolitical structures—and then at the collective level. This also means exploring the spheres in which we have power to lead, teach, or design rules and standards and utilize our influence strategically.

The reflections in this section will help you develop critical self-awareness so that you can participate in building the future you want with an awareness of your own socialization and how that interacts with those around you. It can be very powerful to engage in these reflections with your colleagues and collaborators. We suggest you move through these inquiries thoughtfully and in a radically honest way. These exercises are not meant to shame or blame, but rather to shed light on parts of you that may not always be visible to you. This is not always easy, but it is a necessary part of working toward justice and healing for all. You can utilize the tools from the "Embodied Practices" section to support you staying with the discomfort of this inquiry while engaging with these questions in a resourced and grounded way.

Practicing Change   —KERRI KELLY

In working to understand what roles we have been socialized to play, how we are affected by issues of power and oppression, and how we participate in maintaining or confronting them, it's helpful to make an inventory of our social identities and understand how they operate in our relationships. This is not for the sake of reinforcing categories or hierarchies; it's about understanding them so we can be strategic about how we make the personal, relational, cultural, and systemic changes we need to bring forth balance and equity. Whether we like it or not, we each hold a specific set of social identities related to categories of difference that predispose us to unequal roles in the dynamic system of oppression. These identities are both socially constructed and also very real in terms of the ways people interact with them and assign value based on them. A history of assigned value and ranking has been conferred upon these identities/groups, with male-identified, white, cisgender, straight, nondisabled, and/or wealthy individuals being assigned the most value and rank and those outside of these identities being deemed less worthy and therefore subject to the threat of dominance through violence, exploitation, punishment, and isolation.

The practice of locating ourselves invites us to become more aware of unequal power relations we are a part of so that we can become more skilled in relating across lines of difference and negotiating harm. This can allow our differences to be generative rather than limiting to us. The term *social location* helps people understand the complex and potentially contradictory contexts that shape our different lived experiences.[14] It represents our positionality within society given our social group memberships. Sociologists argue that the social location of an individual profoundly influences who they are and who they become, their interactions with others, and their self-perception, opportunities, and outcomes. It serves to help us better understand the intersections and impacts of our unique lived experiences and the lenses through which we see and interact with the world. From there we can find our right role and responsibility in the work of justice and liberation.

Locate Yourself   —KERRI KELLY

This exercise allows us to explore a spectrum of our identities and where that locates us in relationship to power and privilege so we can better understand how power is structured and how it relates to our identities. This does not represent *who* you are, your personal journey, your life struggles . . . it is simply a representation of how society and dominant culture treat and value you. Our location is never fixed; it is often changing based on context.

Each of us has a social location that reflects our place or position in history and society related to categories of difference (race, gender, class, age, disabilities and abilities, sexual orientation, geographic location, citizenship, etc.). These identities predispose us to unequal roles within the dynamic system of oppression. They are not a reflection of our worth but of the value assigned to the groups we are part of by society. Understanding our social location allows us to become more aware of our unique proximity to power and privilege so that we can more skillfully show up in relationship and take collective action.

Here's how it works:

1. Utilizing the Social Location Wheel on the next page, consider which identities in each category are more privileged (center) and which are more oppressed (margins) in society.

2. Determine your location in each category of difference by placing a dot inside the wheel along the spectrum representing your proximity to privilege or oppression.

3. When you've completed the wheel, draw a line connecting each dot to give you a more holistic sense of your social location as it reflects the aggregate of your identities.

> **NOTE** *Many different sites of privilege and oppression not included in this wheel may feel salient and significant in shaping you and informing your relationships and actions. Feel free to add more spokes to this wheel that better represent aspects of your identity. Categories of difference such as education, language, religion, inherited wealth, and incarceration (among others) are significant indicators of one's location and lived experience and can be substituted or added to the exercise.*

Social Location Wheel

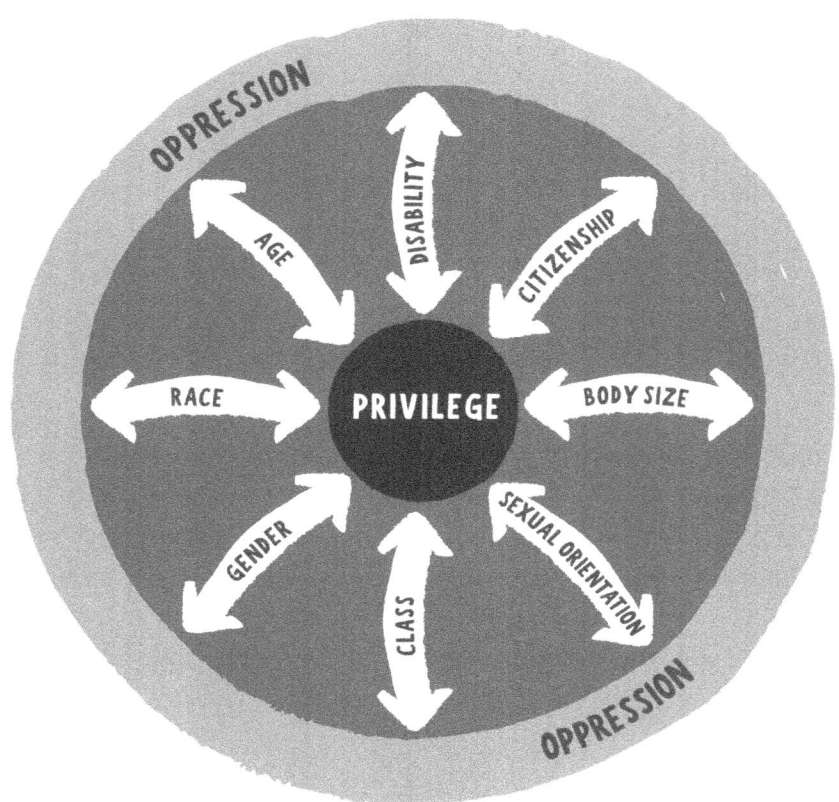

Once you've completed the exercise, consider how your social location informs your role and responsibility in transforming our world into one where everyone can thrive. Consider the many circles and spheres of influence you move inside (professional, familial, etc.) and how you can show up and play your unique role in disrupting, divesting, repairing, or healing spaces. Locating ourselves gives us the awareness to show up in our communities with skill and impact.

Critical Reflection on Self-Identity and Social Location
—TESSA HICKS PETERSON[15]

Reflecting on your self-identity and this notion of social location, consider answering the following prompts alone or with others, in writing or through another contemplative practice.

1. Do the levels of privilege society assigns you as a result of these identity traits correlate with how you view yourself or your experiences in the world?

_____

_____

_____

2. What price do you pay or have others paid for you to stand where you are?

_____

_____

_____

3. What challenges and strengths or insecurities and securities are attached to your different identities?

_____

_____

_____

4. How have these identities shaped the lens with which you view the world and the ways you are treated in the world?

_____

_____

_____

5. Where does privilege show up in your life, explicitly and implicitly?

6. Where does exclusion or discrimination show up in your life, explicitly and implicitly?

7. If you feel guilt, how can you recognize it without being immobilized by it?

8. If you feel anger, how can you use it strategically to make change?

9. Are there ways you dissociate from injustice and oppression (i.e., by going into denial, blame, ignorance, apathy, distraction, numbness, rage, lashing out, or shrinking back)?

10. Provide real examples of what it looks like or could look like to engage in healing or restorative processes over personal or intergenerational oppression you've experienced.

11. Provide real examples of what it looks like (or could look like) to leverage your areas of privilege in the name of peace and justice. What could reparations look like in your own life, family, city?

Embodying Liberation   —ADAPTED FROM AUGUSTO BOAL[16]

This is an exercise that comes from Theatre of the Oppressed, which was developed by Augusto Boal, a Brazilian drama theorist and political activist dedicated to using theater as a means for "rehearsing revolution" with oppressed groups of people. We encourage you to adapt this exercise so that it feels relevant to the specific work you do. The main idea is to attempt to embody what we are hoping to change in the world and what we are hoping to make a reality. You may use the word *oppression* as a general term for what you want to change, and *liberation* to express what you are working toward, or choose your own words—whatever captures what is meaningful to you.

STEP 1: TAKE THE SHAPE OF *OPPRESSION* WITH YOUR BODY.

1. Notice what shape emerges.
2. As you stay with the shape, exaggerate it a little bit; notice how this feels in your body.
3. Notice your thoughts.
4. Exaggerate it a bit more.
5. Stay here for one minute.
6. Shake it off.

STEP 2: TAKE THE SHAPE OF *LIBERATION* WITH YOUR BODY.

1. Notice what shape emerges.
2. As you stay with the shape, exaggerate it a little bit; notice how this feels in your body.
3. Notice your thoughts.
4. Exaggerate it a bit more.
5. Stay here for one minute.
6. Shake it off.

STEP 3: TAKE THE SHAPE OF *OPPRESSION* AND THEN USE FIVE FULL MINUTES TO TRANSITION INTO THE SHAPE OF *LIBERATION*.

1. Don't rush; you can use a timer.
2. Notice your sensations, thoughts, and impulses when you slow it all down.
3. Notice what the transition itself feels like (are there moments of frustration, defeat, excitement, or hope?).

STEP 4: REFLECTION

1. What did you notice about that process?
2. What surprised you?

3. How does embodying these concepts differ from analyzing or discussing them?

4. How might this reveal the challenges that we may encounter in our work toward liberation?

5. Does this exercise reflect any of the dynamics that emerge in the work you are doing or want to do?

Critical Reflection on Personal Motivation
—TESSA HICKS PETERSON

Many of us are motivated to do changemaking work because of our personal experiences struggling with or overcoming abuse or discrimination. In many ways, our gift is in our wounds, and our wounds can become our gifts. This reflection asks you to think about the life experiences that have shaped you and consider how they affect your motivations and actions. It is important that we bring into our awareness these unconscious dynamics so that we can allow our lived experience to be a source of wisdom rather than to cloud our perception and confuse our own internal experience with the external reality. Reflect on the following prompts to deepen your self-awareness around how your motivations may impact your work:

1. What inspires and motivates you to do work around social change?

2. What memories and feelings emerge when you visualize what originally motivated you?

3. Are there ways in which these motivations are connected to your own traumas or wounds and not directly related to the changemaking issue itself?

4. If so, in what ways do any experiences you've personally had still have a grip on your thoughts, behaviors, or emotional reactions today?

5. What can you do to remain conscious of your own healing process so that it can strengthen your work rather than hinder it?

6. What support systems and people can you reach out to in order to support your own healing so you can be sustainable and effective as a changemaker?

PART II

COMMUNITY BUILDING AND CONNECTION

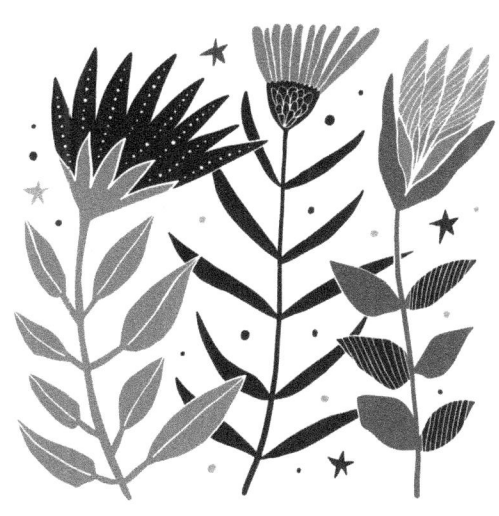

At the heart of the quest for social justice is the right of all people to feel seen, heard, valued, and cared for. It is also about finding ways for our differences to coexist and be celebrated so that everyone has an authentic experience of belonging. Dominant culture often pits our needs against each other and fosters a culture of competition and assimilation rather than inclusivity and belonging. One of the most radical things we can do is build cultures inside our organizations that are nurturing and life affirming for everyone involved, even amid the stress and challenges we are facing.

Community building practices can help us learn how to be together in a way that centers everyone's fullness and humanity. This is new for many of us, which is why being able to be uncomfortable and fumble together is vital. Envisioning a shared intention and creating shared agreements can help lay the groundwork for this type of culture-building work. This includes finding opportunities for folks to engage together in a low-stakes and playful way. When groups are used to only being together amid the stress and urgency of their work, it can wear away at a sense of camaraderie and positive connection. Just like any relationship that doesn't have time and space to refuel its connection, the relationships between people who work together can start to feel tense and frayed if the only time they are interacting is around intense work issues. It might be helpful to think about some of these practices as an organizational "date night" where you agree not to talk about work and focus simply on connecting and finding joy in a non-stressful way. This can fill the well of connection so that people feel more resourced and able to collaborate together so they can deal with stress in a creative and united way.

In many ways, community building practices allow us to embody an inclusive, just, and caring culture, here and now, even when external structures and systems may not. When we create connection, care, well-being, and agency within our own spheres of influence, we are building the world we want in the one we have. Beyond simply surviving oppressive forces, we work toward thriving, knowing that the affirmation of our values, cultures, identities, and well-being is also a form of resistance. By engaging in healing practices collectively, we are able to share in our struggles; find empathy, compassion, and solidarity; build hope, trust, and relationships in which to lift each other up; and together, imagine radical ways in which a better world could operate. We also must remember to create the joy we want in the world we are building. Joy, play, delight, care, and connection are absolutely crucial to changemaking work!

Many of these practices require vulnerability, trust, and patience. They ask us to bring our full selves to the table so we can be in relationships that are authentic and healthy. Doing this work won't always be fast, easy, or comfortable, but remember that discomfort can be a sign of growth. In fact, most growth requires us to move out of our comfort zone! One of the most challenging parts of building a culture of care and connection in our work together is finding ways to be in the uncomfortable process of growth and learning without resorting to shame, blame, conflict, and disconnection. The tools in this workbook can help you stay grounded in the face of discomfort so that you can be discerning about when discomfort is a necessary edge you need to confront in order to grow, or when it is a signal that something is wrong that you need to address.

Remember, the ultimate goal of these practices is to create more ease, creativity, joy, and sustainability in your work and in the world. It's about loving each other in the fullest sense. As Cornel West says, "Justice is what love looks like in public."[1] So, let's bring on the love!

BUILDING BRAVE SPACES

It can take some skill to create spaces where people feel comfortable being authentic and expressive. This section offers some simple yet profound practices that can help create a climate for collaboration that invites the fullness of each of its members in. It begins with some tips on the art of facilitating group processes and includes icebreakers in which participants can move together and share parts of themselves to build a foundation of trust. Such trust is critical to build the container in which a group will be able to eventually navigate harder topics and challenges in their work. With clear communication agreements and listening techniques, facilitating group processes that build a culture of care, mutuality, and collaboration can ignite powerful changemaking work.

Effective Facilitation   —TESSA HICKS PETERSON

One key to being successful in collective changemaking work is thoughtful facilitation of community building and connection practices. We recognize that group dynamics can be complex and some issues deserve outside facilitation support. Sometimes groups hire an outside facilitator to take them through certain exercises and processes, but for many people, it's more realistic to have those inside the organization play that role. It is a good idea to make sure in-house facilitators have studied and practiced the techniques of strong facilitation. The following provides context and key components for effective facilitation.

The root of facilitation is the attempt to make the process at hand *facile*, that is, easy. A facilitator helps guide the group, keep them on task, resolve conflict, and ensure that the goals and intentions of the group are met. A facilitator helps create spaces in which all can feel safe, respected, present, committed, and open to the work at hand so they can share candid thoughts about the given topic and show up fully. With skillful guidance, such group work can become a place of deep connection, discovery, and effective action. It is also a place where strong community trust is cultivated so that the group can withstand the inevitable conflicts that arise without being disassembled (in spirit or actuality) by hard conversations and decisions.

So that a facilitator's own feelings or opinions don't interrupt their role of guiding others in dialogue, they must be aware of their own positionality, values, communication style, biases, and triggers. Cofacilitation with a trusted partner is a great option. It can promote diverse representations of ways to lead, while also offering support so that it's not on one person to hold the whole process on their own. You can also share leadership responsibilities among group members, or rotate facilitators and take turns anchoring particular exercises and processes.

Here are some key components for effective facilitation:

Energizing: Bringing ease, warmth, and connection into the room through icebreakers, mindfulness moments, or pair-share activities.

Guiding: Creating an arc to the experience, from introducing people and topics to supplying prompts, reflections, debriefs, and concluding remarks or next steps.

Active listening and clarifying: Listening carefully, clarifying misunderstandings, asking follow-up questions, modeling being unafraid of silence.

Managing group dynamics: Overseeing time limits, agenda aims, equal group participation, and safety for all participants; directly addressing conflict or harm; and keeping the group on task.

Summarizing: Reflecting back what's been said and weaving distinct threads together.

Community Agreements   —TESSA HICKS PETERSON[2]

One way to create a safe- and brave-enough space in which people can navigate discomfort successfully for learning and growth to occur is by creating *community agreements*. Community agreements can also be thought of as group norms that we want to establish to build a culture of inclusion, care, honesty, and respect. Creating these can also lay the groundwork for compassionate and effective communication. Clear agreements can support work meetings, educational spaces, community organizing spaces, therapeutic spaces, and even one-on-one interactions. Adapt them to fit any situation you are in where you want to support healthy communication. The most meaningful way to do this collaboratively is by inviting everyone to share an agreement they'd like to bring into the space. When people offer their own suggestions, they are more invested in being accountable to them.

The following list provides some suggested agreements that can help create spaces in which people feel safe and supported to speak their truth and listen generously.

Take a breath before responding: The more grounded we are when we speak, the more skillful our communication will be. To do the best that you can, settle yourself before you speak in order to respond mindfully rather than react impulsively.

Hold space for multiple truths and perspectives: You may hear ideas that may be new or different to you and opinions with which you may disagree. Try to take in new information with curiosity. Remember that you are likely in a setting with people who all have a good intention and are doing the best they can. Engage contemplative, embodied listening, which means being open, present, and mindful of what is being said, listening deeply, and responding thoughtfully.

Speak from the "I": Speak from your own personal experiences and avoid judging the thoughts or experiences of others. Use I-statements such as *"I feel . . ."* or "In my experience. . . ." Avoid "You should" or "We all know" statements and generalizations of any kind.

Share "air time": Help create a space in which everyone can speak. No one, however, is obligated to speak. If you tend to speak a lot, make sure you are also listening generously. If you tend to not speak, lean into bringing your voice to the conversation if you sense it would support you or the group. Recognize how your positionality often impacts how much air time you tend to take.

Attend to both intention and impact: If you say something that hurts someone else, even if it was not your intention, attend to the impact rather than doubling down on your intention. We are all learning. Sharing context around intention may be helpful, but taking accountability around impact is vital.

Call in rather than call out: Ask engaging questions and call people in to learn with you rather than calling them out about where you think they are wrong (recognize that harsh judgment and shaming don't move us toward understanding).

Movements/Opposites —ADAPTED FROM AUGUSTO BOAL

Icebreakers are methods for inviting people to connect in a low-stakes situation in order to build enough trust to connect in deeper, more vulnerable ways. They can also be used to nurture connection when a group is used to only engaging with each other in intense and urgent situations. Finding ways to be settled together allows groups to build the resilience to face stressful situations with more skill and less conflict. It also helps build flexibility into our interactions so we can move from being in a mode of urgency, when that is needed, to creativity, when that is called for. Ultimately, this is groundwork for building the trustworthy relationships and meaningful community a group needs to support any transformative work they will do together.

The purpose of the "Movements/Opposites" icebreaker exercise is to help us let go of perfectionism, jostle our senses, and loosen up together.[3] It's meant to be silly! Please pick the exercises that are accessible to the people in the space. If folks have mobility restrictions, work with the first set only and don't require people to move about the room. Feel free to make up any prompts that are appropriate for your group.

1. Designate a facilitator. They will shout out a command the group then follows.

2. Instruct the group to move about the room randomly.

SET 1

When I say, "yell your name!" wave your arms.

When I say, "wave your arms!" yell your name.

Repeat each instruction and watch to see if the group remembers to do the other instruction that you gave them.

Do this a few times alternating instructions. Then add in the next set.

SET 2

When I say, "spin around," take a bow.

When I say, "take a bow," spin around.

Do this a few times then add in the first set of instructions occasionally.

[The group is usually giggling and laughing at this point.]

OPTIONAL: ADD ANOTHER SET.

When I say, "cluck like a chicken!" do an exaggerated yawn.

When I say, "yawn!" cluck like a chicken.

Repeat and add in the other sets.

OPTIONAL: REFLECT AFTERWARD AS A GROUP:

How did it feel to do the opposite of what is being asked of you?

How did it feel to make mistakes?

How did it feel to be ridiculous together?

Why might it be important for us to practice breaking perfectionist habits and loosening up together?

Embodied Listening   —SCARLETT DUARTE

Most of us have unconsciously internalized a culture of white supremacy in our organizations, where listening is not prioritized and we end up reproducing toxic behaviors in the spaces where we seek to dismantle those things. By not listening to our colleagues and community members, we risk enabling a climate of defensiveness and power hoarding that prevents others from equally participating and feeling appreciated. Barriers to effective communication can disrupt information flow, interpersonal relationships, quality work, and vision. Therefore, a deep commitment to listening and nonverbal communication can foster proactive engagement toward conflict resolution, employee morale, and better leadership.

One way we can do this is by engaging *embodied listening*—listening with our whole body, which is a kind of deep listening in which we are fully present with others. We can accomplish this by maintaining eye contact or by using verbal cues of engagement and mirroring. We can also give someone space and encourage them to share their experience fully without interrupting, analyzing, giving advice, or judging. We also want to avoid shifting the topic to ourselves, or trying to be helpful before help is asked for (which may require us to suspend a sense of self-importance or ego). The purpose of embodied listening is for listeners to strive to understand and hold space for the speaker without any interruption and for the speaker to feel fully heard and held in the conversation.

You can try embodied listening anytime you find yourself in a conversation. You might also deliberately set up a time to practice with someone. If you do that, choose a specific topic around which you would like to feel heard or hear someone else. Designate a time, place, and length of conversation that feels good to both parties. You should make sure each person has a separate time to speak, so arrange the plan accordingly. You can set a timer or allow the conversation to unfold organically. Try using the tools in this workbook related to interoception and self-regulation to stay in your body and remain grounded and present so you can listen with your whole being. After the exercise, reflect on this experience with these questions:

1. Are you aware of direct bodily sensations as you listen?

2. Where do you experience these sensations as you listen?

3. Are you engaged in a daydream as you listen?

4. Are you aware of emotions as you listen?

5. Do you feel able to truly listen and hold the speaker?

6. Are you aware of direct bodily sensations as you speak?

7. Where do you experience sensation as you speak?

8. Do you feel heard and held by the listener?

9. Are you aware of emotions as you speak?

10. Is there anything else you want to share about this experience?

11. Are there specific times and spaces at/in which you might imagine integrating this practice into your work or your community that would be helpful?

12. Are there additional practices you want to draw on to fortify your ability to embody more awareness when you listen and when you speak?

Concentric Circles   —TESSA HICKS PETERSON[4]

This exercise can be used as a community-building icebreaker as well as a chance to practice embodied listening.

Ask participants to count off one, two, one, two . . . , until they have all been assigned a one or a two. Ask all the "ones" to form a circle with room between them (standing or sitting in chairs). Then ask the "twos" to form a circle *around* the ones. At this point, ask the inner circle to turn outward so that the inner and outer circles face each other, creating concentric circles. Now pairs should be formed between individuals in the inner and outer circles. Make sure pairs are close enough to hear each other well and let them know they will be asked a question that each person will have two minutes to answer. The aim is for partners to practice embodied listening when the other is talking, which means making space for the speaker to feel fully heard and not responding with input, advice, or one's own stories. Keep time and ask partners to change turns speaking at the two-minute mark. After both partners have shared for two minutes each, have the outside circle move clockwise one space to create a new partner pair and ask a new question. After you have asked some or all of the suggested questions, facilitate a debrief about what participants learned, felt, and gained from this experience (highlighting the impact of the intentional, embodied listening component) and how it uncovered some of who they are and the aims of their coming together.

Suggested concentric circles prompts include the following:

1. What is the story of your name (first, middle, last, or nickname)?
2. Where are you from (geographically, politically, culturally, spiritually)?
3. What communities do you belong to and which feels most important right now?
4. What price do you pay (and have others paid) for you to be where you are today?
5. What inspires you to do this work?
6. What keeps you in this work when it gets hard?
7. Where do you find joy in this work?
8. Where do you find rage in this work?
9. Where do you find refueling/restoration in this work?

Active Listening   —HALA KHOURI

Embodied listening can lay the groundwork for *active listening*, which invites in another layer of communication with the goal of letting the other person know that you hear them and are trying to understand their point of view or experience. This involves engaging with the speaker throughout the conversation in ways that signal to them that you are listening explicitly through your body language, tone of voice, and words. If we're not first aware of what is happening inside our own body, mind, and heart, it can be very hard to actually listen when someone is speaking because we can be distracted by our own internal experience. Active listening requires us to set aside our own need to be heard (for now) and focus fully on trying to understand what the other person is saying. In situations when we encounter conflict, active listening can diffuse or deescalate tension and lay the groundwork for an authentic two-way conversation.

ACTIVE LISTENING IS

- Staying self-regulated while you listen. Practice being grounded, present, curious, and open.
- Mirroring back what the other person said to you.
    - Use their exact words ("I hear that made you really upset").
    - Or use other words and clarifying meaning ("You said that that meeting made you want to quit; are you feeling angry because of what was said?").
    - Mirror using your body language and tones; otherwise, people can feel talked down to. Try to match their energy, but not in a way that escalates the conversation.
- Asking clarifying questions.
    - "Can you tell me more about what that was like for you?"
    - "Can you say more about that?"

ACTIVE LISTENING IS NOT

- Giving advice.
- Analyzing.
- Sympathizing.
- Talking about your own experience.
- Agreeing or disagreeing with the person (they may be saying something that you completely disagree with, but they still need to feel heard in order to be able to listen to another perspective).

When both speakers in a dialogue feel that they have been actively listened to as they speak their truth, it can create the container and willingness to stretch themselves into greater empathy, understanding, and a shared commitment to finding common ground. Active listening can lay the groundwork for effective conflict resolution.

> NOTE *It is important to recognize the various power dynamics that exist between people and how they can impact communication. The person with more power in their role (i.e., supervisor, boss, executive director) always has the greater responsibility to explicitly try to create a safe atmosphere for communication and feedback. We also need to consider current and historical power dynamics based on identity that may be at play (i.e., between a white person and a person of color). It's for this reason that reflection on our own socialization and positionality has to be part of the process of community care and collaboration.*

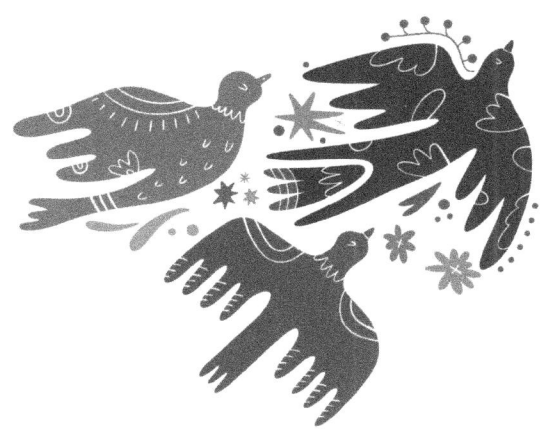

FOSTERING CREATIVE CONNECTIONS

Having space to be playful and creative together can sometimes bring the heart and soul back to our collective work. When groups are caught in the urgency and exhaustion of the daily grind it can strain relationships and undermine effective collaboration. These exercises can serve as a group "pause" to get grounded together in an embodied and creative way. They can stoke the fires of creativity and reinvigorate relationships so that we can reconnect to a sense of joy, hope, and faith in our shared vision.

Breathing and Moving as a Collective
—BELOVED COMMUNITIES NETWORK

Exploring how to move and breathe together as a collective can deepen the clarity of our vision, our shared purpose, and the relationship that we have with each other. Through embodied practices, we are building our muscles to align with our values into movement and organizational spaces. This embodied exercise is intended to teach us to breathe, to feel our individual bodies, and to move as a collective.

In a circle facing inward, standing or seated, have each person place their feet on the floor and make a connection to everything that is underneath and supporting them. Guide them through the following practice.

Focus on the spine and parts of the body that hold your body together. Interlock your hands and guide them down to your belly. While inhaling, stretch your arms slowly up and over your head. Stretch the core. Exhale and let your arms flow down back to the sides until your hands are touching in front of your body. Cross your arms at the heart to gather more space and return to the inhaling stretch, lifting your arms up, then the exhaling movement to bring your arms back down. Repeat this practice two to three times. Go at your own pace.

As you do this, notice each other and notice who is the closest to your pace and rhythm. Intentionally line up with this individual so that your movements mirror each other. Think about what it feels like to align yourself with that person. Try doing the activity a second time, this time intentionally working together so that your movements and the pace of breaths sync up with another's from beginning to end, and so you become present to that experience of physical alignment. At the end of the breathing and moving exercise, reflect together on how it felt to match each other's breath and to move as a collective. Consider together: How might this translate into aligning values, actions, and strategies in organizational and movement work?

Music as Connective Tissue —TESSA HICKS PETERSON

As Stevie Wonder sings in "Sir Duke," music is a language we all understand. Music has always been an inspiration and guide for social movements and community building, so imagine all the ways you can use it in your collaborations. You can:

- Sing together.
- Chant together.
- Write a song together.
- Take out some instruments and just jam together.
- Write down the lyrics of old protest songs, and as you play each song, gather as a group to analyze their meaning and the impact they had on people and movements.
- Ask everyone to contribute a song to a shared playlist that they feel best embodies the changes they are advocating for or the feeling changemaking gives them and listen to it in your work, in your protests, in your dance parties!

"We Are From" Group Poem —TESSA HICKS PETERSON[5]

This practice aims to foster creative connections and cohesion across diverse groups of people working together. It was adapted from a version experienced in a prison education workshop.

1. Instruct participants to work individually to write a poem about where they're from. Start each sentence with the line, "I am from . . . ," and ask participants to fill in the

rest of the sentence with vivid imagery, bringing to life what it feels like, looks like, smells like, tastes like, or sounds like to be where they are from. Invite participants to relinquish nervousness around poetic cadence or spelling—anyone can do this! Remind them that being specific and vulnerable helps us connect with our own experience and with each other.

2. After ten minutes of individual writing, return to the large group and ask each person to share their poem while everyone else actively listens and takes notes on any vivid imagery that struck them from someone else's poem. (Remember to encourage participants to take risks, but always make it optional to share.)

3. Following each sharing of a poem, invite another participant to share one image or line that stayed with them from someone else's poem and why.

4. Ask each poet to choose their favorite line from their own poem.

5. Invite everyone to create a circle together wherein each person takes a turn and reads aloud their chosen line from their poem, one after another, until everyone has shared.

6. Ask the group to do that again, but this time, ask participants to change the first pronoun in their line from "I" to "We," so each line reads "We are from . . ." Each person's offered line should follow directly after the last one so it becomes one collective "We Are From" poem.

7. After the final version of the "We Are From" poem has been recited, follow up with a group debrief exploring both the process and the product of the activity and if/how participants understand the concepts and each other differently as a result of engaging in this form of individual and group expression.

8. Close the activity by reminding participants that this poem can only be created with this particular group of individuals, today. It binds the group together, even though personal experiences are distinct. Discuss together in what ways the arts have served as a vehicle for personal healing, collective empowerment, and community building.

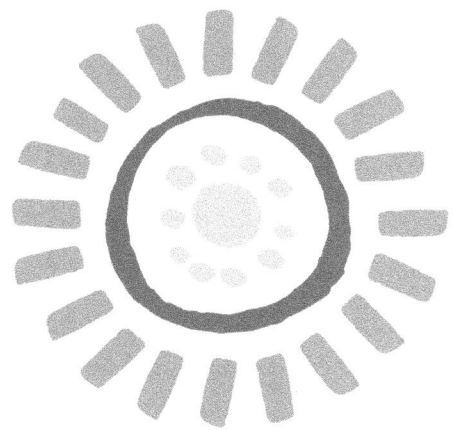

STRENGTHENING OUR ORGANIZATIONS

All too often, organizations fall apart or become ineffective because of breakdowns in the relationships. Strong organizations are grounded in relational practices that allow people inside the organization to show up in their fullness, build trust, and handle conflict well. Organizations also need to be explicit about their values and do their best to create a culture that is a reflection of these values. The practices in this section are meant to become a central part of organizational culture and to be used consistently. Culture building is like brushing your teeth; we do it daily as a ritual and a habit.

Organizational Wholeness   —KAZU HAGA

What does it mean for a community to create space for everyone to be able to show up whole? What can an organization implement to let people bring "all of themselves" into a space? We must understand that well-being is every person's birthright; it shouldn't have to be earned, and it is essential to supporting everyone in a workplace. On an individual level, this might look like allowing people to bring their animals with them to work, or giving each person a small budget to decorate a part of the shared space in a way that they would like. On an organizational level, it could look like building relational and resiliency practices into the schedule and overall flow—something as simple as a shared potluck meal once a week or engaging in some of this workbook's practices. Here are some simple ideas of how to explicitly value, in word and action, organizational wholeness:

Porous Walls: When an organization takes its work seriously, it can't limit its concerns to the boundaries of the organization. Support each person's hobbies and passions. This might mean allowing each person to volunteer for a different organization one day each month as part of their staff time or the organization hosting a fundraiser for a different group each month.

Opening Silence: Begin each meeting with a few minutes of silence, allowing people to ground themselves and transition from whatever they may have been working on before. You might be surprised at how big of an impact this small practice can have!

Check-Ins: We live in a world where, in most cases, the question "How are you?" is not a genuine inquiry. We are not expecting the person to actually take a moment to check in with themselves and respond honestly. It can be a simple and generous act to gift each person with a few minutes to share something meaningful about themselves. If they run out of things to say, allow them to sit in silence and see if something else emerges. Sometimes the intimacy of a small group allows more to emerge so check-ins can also be done in pairs or small groups. Simple prompts or structures may support a genuine check-in. Here are some examples:

- Share three words that describe how you are feeling right now.
- If your life right now was a song, what would the title be?
- What's the weather inside? (Use actual weather descriptions to describe your internal landscape!)
- Share with us a rose (something beautiful in your life), bud (something new and still developing in your life), and thorn (something you are struggling with).
- What are you hoping to get out of this meeting?

Appreciation Circles: Go around in a circle and have each person name one specific thing that they are appreciating that is happening in the group's workspace. Or offer a prompt such as "Who was the last person that you appreciated out loud, and why?" Regular practices in appreciation begin to build a culture of appreciation, which can foster respect, belonging, and connection.

Closing Check-In: End meetings by asking a simple prompt, such as "What is one thing you appreciated in this meeting?" or "What is one thing that you want to keep sitting with and exploring from our work together?"

Organizational Resilience   —HALA KHOURI

There are many creative ways to build embodiment, reflection, regulation, and connection practices into organizations and collectives. Doing so can help create the conditions that can handle conflict and support resilient, authentic communication. These practices, like the following examples, can have large results when done consistently. They don't have to take a long time (unless you want them to).

DURING MEETINGS

1. Light a candle, put flowers on the table, put on music, provide fidget toys, or encourage doodling by providing paper and markers . . . do something to make the space feel inviting, creative, and accessible to multiple ways of learning, connecting, and being present.

2. Start with grounding, breathing, or a meditation practice (see Part I of this book for ideas on specific exercises you can do).

3. Do a brief check-in (see the previous "Organizational Wholeness" practices).

4. If it's a long meeting, give people opportunities to stand, stretch, and move around; to take snack or water breaks; to use the bathroom; or to get a moment of fresh air.

5. End with a quick check-out process.

   a. What is one useful takeaway from this meeting?

   b. What is one question you still have?

DURING THE WORKDAY

1. Encourage real lunch breaks for people to restore and refuel. Suggest getting away from the computer and doing something restorative.

2. Encourage community lunches where people sit together to eat without talk about work (this can even happen virtually).

3. Take meetings while walking together.

4. Celebrate birthdays, special holidays, and accomplishments. Any chance to celebrate and intentionally ignite joy should be embraced!

ORGANIZATIONAL RETREATS

1. When possible, a retreat with the intention of building community and nurturing connections and creativity can offer a reset or a space in which to deepen relationships and camaraderie. These moments for connection and restoration are especially important during times of great stress, conflict, or despair.

2. If you have greenspace nearby or even a house or other organizational space someone will let you use, retreat into a new environment and see how that inspires new ideas and connections.

3. If going away to a different location is not possible, consider finding a way to create a nurturing experience inside the walls (or digital rooms) of your organization. Create a two- or three-hour "retreat" where folks do a variety of exercises suggested in this workbook, eat together, vision together, and so on. If you have funds to bring in an external facilitator, doing so can support the process and relinquish established leadership roles as well.

GROUP SHARING PRACTICES

A STRONG WAY to build community is to speak together in an intimate circle dialogue. Circles of storytelling, ritual, and governance have been a part of cultures worldwide for millennia. A practice called *council* has its roots in many different Native American and First Nations cultures and has been respectfully adapted for use in the fields of mediation, restorative justice, education, and others. In a council, people sit in a circle so they can connect in a ritualized way. The group passes around a talking piece such as a stone, stick, or special object, and whoever has the piece can speak. Everyone else simply listens without commentary. In some circles, people use their time to check in and share how they are doing. Sometimes the group sets a particular theme and folks respond to a specific question or prompt. There are three main guidelines for people to follow in a council circle: speak from the heart, speak lean, and honor one speaker at a time. Council is one format you can utilize to create a space for group conversation and connection. Having some structure around group conversations is important so that everyone who wants to speak can speak; this is also a way to encourage deep listening. This may sound simple, but it can be quite profound and has been used as a sacred practice for generations.

It can also be important to give people the option to connect in smaller groups. Some people don't feel comfortable sharing in a large group and will only open up in a circle of two or three other people at a time. Depending on what your intention is, offering a space where people break into small groups can be a powerful way to foster connection among people working together. Consider how people are divided up—for example, sometimes it makes sense to group people with others that they work intimately with, but at other times it can be important to allow folks who may not normally connect to be together. This can be a powerful way to build a sense of community and strengthen collaborations.

Practicing Generative Conflict   —KAZU HAGA

Difficult conversations are important and necessary to have, especially if you want to facilitate conflict in a way that can be generative. The process for navigating conflict shared here is adapted from Nonviolent Communication (NVC) teacher and activist Miki Kashtan. For generative conflict to occur, three conditions must be present: structure, strong relationships, and skills of the people in the dialogue. Together these can create a space for open communication, deep listening processes for meaningful conversations, and greater understanding of relationship building.

When thinking about "structure," consider if there is a setting that supports a brave space for all involved in the conversation. This can include a clearly laid-out agenda, a clear system or formula for how communication will happen including who will speak first, and the integration of approaches and tools that help to create a strong container. (See the "Group Sharing Practices" box for some ideas on how to set up the conversation as well as the other practices in this section that can support the creation of a strong container.)

With relationships, you want to assess how well the parties involved in a conflict know each other and how much trust exists between them in that moment—knowing that trust is dynamic and can change based on current dynamics and circumstances.

In regard to skill, you want to consider things like how grounded a person is when they are in conflict, how well they are able to listen to different perspectives and express their true feelings, their ability to speak from their personal experiences, and whether they have taken any past trainings on conflict engagement, nonviolent communication, or any other relevant skill sets. You also want to consider if a facilitator is needed to help guide the conversation, what kind of skill set that facilitator needs, and who that person should be (so that all parties feel safe, seen, and able to trust and engage in the process).

Before navigating a conflict, consider the following questions:

- How much structure is there? Is everyone clear on the plans and intention for the dialogue? Is there a clear agenda?
- How strong are the relationships in the room? How much trust is there?
- How much skill is present in the room in terms of people's abilities to participate in difficult discussions skillfully?

If any of these things are not strong enough to hold the conflict and facilitate it in a generative way, then the work becomes about building these resources first. This can take time but is well worth it because it sets you up to deal with other conflicts should they arise. Every organization and collaboration is different, but here are some ideas to guide your process:

- If you lack structure, consider using a talking piece, holding a talking circle, creating a highly structured agenda, or utilizing tools like Nonviolent Communication.
- If you sense that the relationships are not strong enough, it may be supportive for your organization to host more team-building activities like having meals together, playing games, or sharing each other's stories and getting to know each other outside of a work context.
- If you are lacking in skills for conflict engagement, you can bring in a skilled facilitator, attend a workshop together, or even engage in a shared study of conflict resolution.

Conflict is the spirit of the relationship asking itself to deepen. Practicing the skills to make conflict generative opens the possibilities for a culture of accountability, compassion, and transparency for communities to build on harm.

Consider how you might build a culture that can hold conflict and allow it to be generative. This is no easy task and asks us to often reevaluate many of our foundational assumptions and practices. What can you do to strengthen relationships, and build skills around communication, accountability, and self-responsibility? What skills and structures can you develop to facilitate conflict so that it becomes generative, not extractive or destructive?

Value Explicit Systems   —KAZU HAGA

Values guide actions and systems. Individuals, communities, and organizations operate on value systems that guide their structure, processes, and operations, but the value systems themselves are not often spelled out. An *implicit value system* is one that nobody (or very few) in the organization has formally agreed to. These are often systems that the majority has been socialized into, ones that have been passed down by the dominant paradigm. An *explicit system* is one where everyone in the organization has talked about the system and how their own values align with their work and has agreed upon how they are going to do things together. It is important to recognize whether members of the organization have a voice in building organizations and systems that reflect their values and purpose.

Ultimately, the goal is to collaborate and cultivate organizations working toward the shared vision that their members have, and to produce a culture and practices that resemble the world that folks seek to build now. The purpose of this exercise is to examine current organizational structures, policies, processes, and cultures, and to determine whether they resonate and align with the collective values. Think about the examined and unexamined values that influence the organizational culture. How might it be possible to embody the values that the collective wants in our existing structure?

Decision-Making: Who makes decisions? Who gives input? What is the process? Do individuals feel safe and included to participate and share their opinions?

Information Flow: How does information flow? In what direction? What information is shared? Who has access to information?

Resource Flow: What resources exist? What kinds of resources are honored? How are they distributed? Is the organization's budget transparent, including everyone's salaries?

Feedback Systems: Who gives feedback? Who receives it? When and why does feedback happen?

Conflict Engagement: Who do people go to when there is conflict? How are conflicts resolved?

Reflect together on this process and what needs to be shifted to move toward greater value alignment. (More relationship and trust building? Commitments to practices of self and community care? Clearer processes of communication and program building? Different forms of defining and assessing "success"?)

Consider what is working well and what are the challenges or gaps that block systems from aligning with organizational values and purpose. Create clear strategies for how to build toward shared goals.

CREATING THE CONDITIONS FOR CARE

IF YOU ARE in a senior position or any position of power, it is vital to support personal and collective care practices as well as recognize how you and your organization can be accountable to power imbalances and inequities. It is also critical to think about how to be in alignment with the values and principles of community care and justice in your operations in terms of workload, workflow, communication, and overall organizational policies. This includes vacation time, sick days, organizational climate, governance, decision-making, and conflict resolution protocols. When the staff of an organization feels unsupported by senior management, attempts by management to offer practices for resilience can feel like (and often are) attempts to put the responsibility on the workers to figure out how to be well inside of an organization that is actively creating barriers to wellness or empowerment.[6]

For folks who do not have institutional power, collective care practices are vital in coping with and pushing against the current conditions. These practices of mutuality and support can also help individuals to not internalize or blame themselves for how they are feeling inside of a system that doesn't support their well-being.

PART III

COLLECTIVE IMAGINING

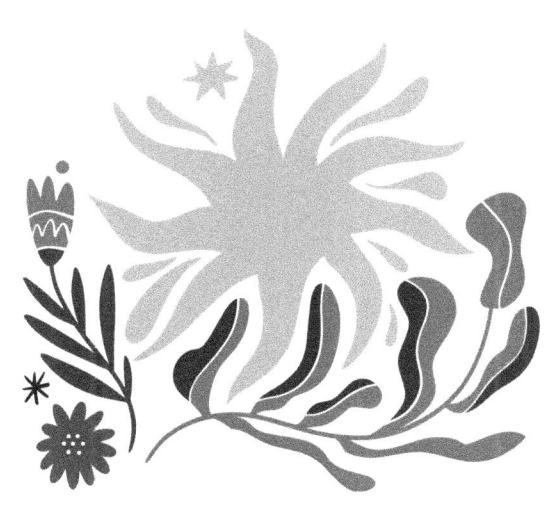

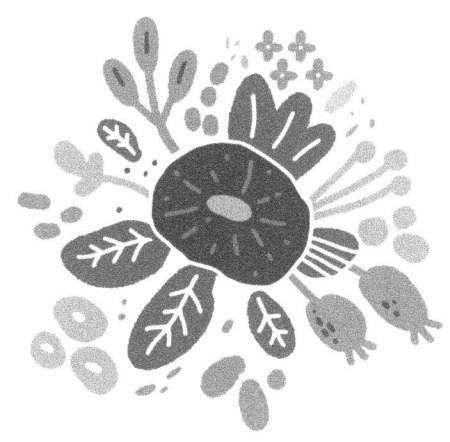

DREAMING TOGETHER

Robin D. G. Kelley's concept of "freedom dreams" essentially connects what is (what we see with our own two eyes) and what could be (what we perceive through the creative and critical lens of our third eye).[1] We acknowledge and analyze the various crises of our times—injustice, illness, greed, violence—and radically imagine a world that will better attend to our needs and uplift our interdependence and well-being instead. What kinds of language will we use to describe and create a world centering healing and justice? What images, visions, principles, and values do we want to guide such dreams? How might we translate these dreams into shared strategies and action plans? This section aims to inspire just this kind of reflection and visioning of the well and just world you and your collaborators might imagine.

To make long-term and effective change in the various sectors we are working in, we must begin by naming the unjust and unwell systems in our society—and the norms, behaviors, and ideologies that undergird them. To transform them, we must truly understand and get free from the harmful individual and collective paradigms within which we are deeply embedded. We must slow down enough to really see, reflect on, and analyze them, and then sit with whatever rage, grief, surprise, sorrow, regret, shame, or immobilization may arise. We must lean into any discomfort this process brings up—accompany it, honor it, and learn from it in order to grow from it. Contemplative, critical reflection is key here. We may be tempted to rush to a sophisticated analysis that pulls us away from our hearts and into our heads too quickly due to the vulnerability this work asks of us. Or we may want to rage against the unjust and unwell systems but know that if we do so, we will not have the energy we need to imagine and build just and well ones instead.

To embody a real transformation, we have to be willing to show up a bit naked and raw and defrost the freeze response of holding trauma at the individual and collective levels so we can imagine that another way is possible. Beyond fostering awareness and change on an individual level, we also need to practice critical reflection collectively in order to develop roadmaps and transformative strategies for systems change. Once we engage together in reflection of what it is we want to dismantle, harness, and build anew, we can courageously disrupt toxic systems and move toward radical imaginations of liberatory futures.

In order to create a better world, we must first radically imagine her into being. Radical imagination challenges the foundation of what has been normalized and invites us to question and reimagine beyond what we've ever known. Radical imagination shakes the very foundation of what we have been told are intractable parts of our reality. This imagining is risky, it's destabilizing, and it uproots things we thought were necessary. Without radical imagination, we are left only with what we currently know, which limits what could be. adrienne maree brown reminds us that the world that we live in now—its systems, structures, norms, and expectations—was imagined by those who came before us but did not include all of us. What can we imagine, and then create together, that would ensure that liberty and justice for all was an actual lived experience for all? What repair and healing do we need in order to move beyond surviving and into thriving as we build the world we want? If we do not attempt to practice those values and qualities now, we set ourselves up to reproduce old harms under new leadership.

So, what is this world we dream of? What would it look like, feel like, and sound like there? To have our needs met. To live in peace. To matter. To belong. To be whole. To be cared for. To love and be loved. These things are at the root of the world we deserve and need. To create it, we must enact it with each other until the systems we are part of also reflect it.

This section is a tapestry of exercises, musings, and reflections to inspire you and your comrades to imagine and create together. Sometimes we can jump right into imagining a world of peace, liberation, and well-being, and other times we need to sit first with our grief, rage, and ruminations of what we want to tear down or change before we build. We need both processes! The practices at the start of this workbook can help create the conditions for this imagining to be possible and accessible. Without community-care practices and self-regulation, making space for radical imagination can feel impossible when we are in the fight energy of urgency and survival. Discerning the appropriate community practices and responses based on the circumstances of the moment is important. As one of our collaborators, Nkem Ndefo, explains:

There is a certain fight energy that is needed to dismantle the interlocking systems of oppression. The spirit is urgent, confrontational, and destructive. And it is necessary to interrupt harm. However useful for protection and subversion, this fight energy comes with its own dangers when employed in situations that either don't warrant a fight reaction or ask for a more nuanced response . . . This fight energy is very different from the spirit we need to reimagine liberatory worlds where we thrive. It is more than imagining but rather, as my coconspirators at Healing Justice London say, *rehearsing freedoms*—being and relating to one another in ways that sustainably create equity, support interdependence, celebrate difference, nurture creativity, savor pleasure, and provide nourishing rest. Dreaming and building are spacious and generative processes where we need to be able to hold multiple complexities and remain settled enough in our bodies to connect to our interiority without letting our perspectives and needs eclipse those of others.[2]

"Dreaming and building" processes are uplifted through shared creativity and playfulness, which also help us remember our interconnectedness with all things. Encouraging play and radical imagination is absolutely crucial if we are to develop new ideas and ways of thinking, innovating, and problem-solving the social, racial, political, and ecological crises of our times. To radically alter the norms of violence, domination, and exclusion that are reflected in so many spheres of our lives, we need to support means for both our rest and our exuberant energy, both our restorative practices and our creative and radically imaginative practices. Inspiring play and imagination can look any number of ways, according to the time, setting, and intention. Consider doing an embodied practice or meditation before engaging in some of these exercises. You want your mind, body, and heart in a curious and open space![3]

What Is and What Could Be   —TESSA HICKS PETERSON

McKinsey's Three Horizons framework is a useful starting point for reflecting on our current system and practices. This framework calls first for an analysis of the key characteristics of the prevailing system; second, for an exploration of the values, cultures, laws, and events that led to it; and third, for an explanation of why we believe it's not fit for its purpose and is failing. Evaluating *what is* helps us then imagine *what could be*. This analysis is an important endeavor to undertake as an individual and with fellow changemakers.

Reflect on the following questions in any number of ways—perhaps through journal-writing responses or by engaging in contemplative reflection; maybe you can explore these through theater and embodied interpretations or as questions you share during a retreat for people to reflect on individually or explore in small groups. This is not a quick fix or simple worksheet to fill out; this is an invitation into a longer process of critical analysis, deep reflection, and collective imagining.

Prompts can include:

1. Where do you see this system/institution/organization we are a part of failing and how are you impacted by it?

2. What toxic norms have you become adjusted and conditioned to that should be questioned?

3. Where do you see this system thriving and having a positive impact?

4. What assets and strengths do you want to harness?

5. What can you dream up that would better suit your visions of a just and well world?

6. What are the key characteristics of a just and well world and what would it look like and feel like to be in this world?

7. What history, values, and culture are embedded within it?

8. What actors are already working on this liberatory future and who can be collaborated with so the new system scales and spreads?

9. Which assumptions will be most challenged by this change?

_____

_____

_____

10. Who are most vulnerable to these emerging changes?

_____

_____

_____

11. Who are most strengthened by these emerging changes?

_____

_____

_____

12. How will we know when we've reached our visions of a just and well world?[4]

_____

_____

_____

Beloved Communities Network

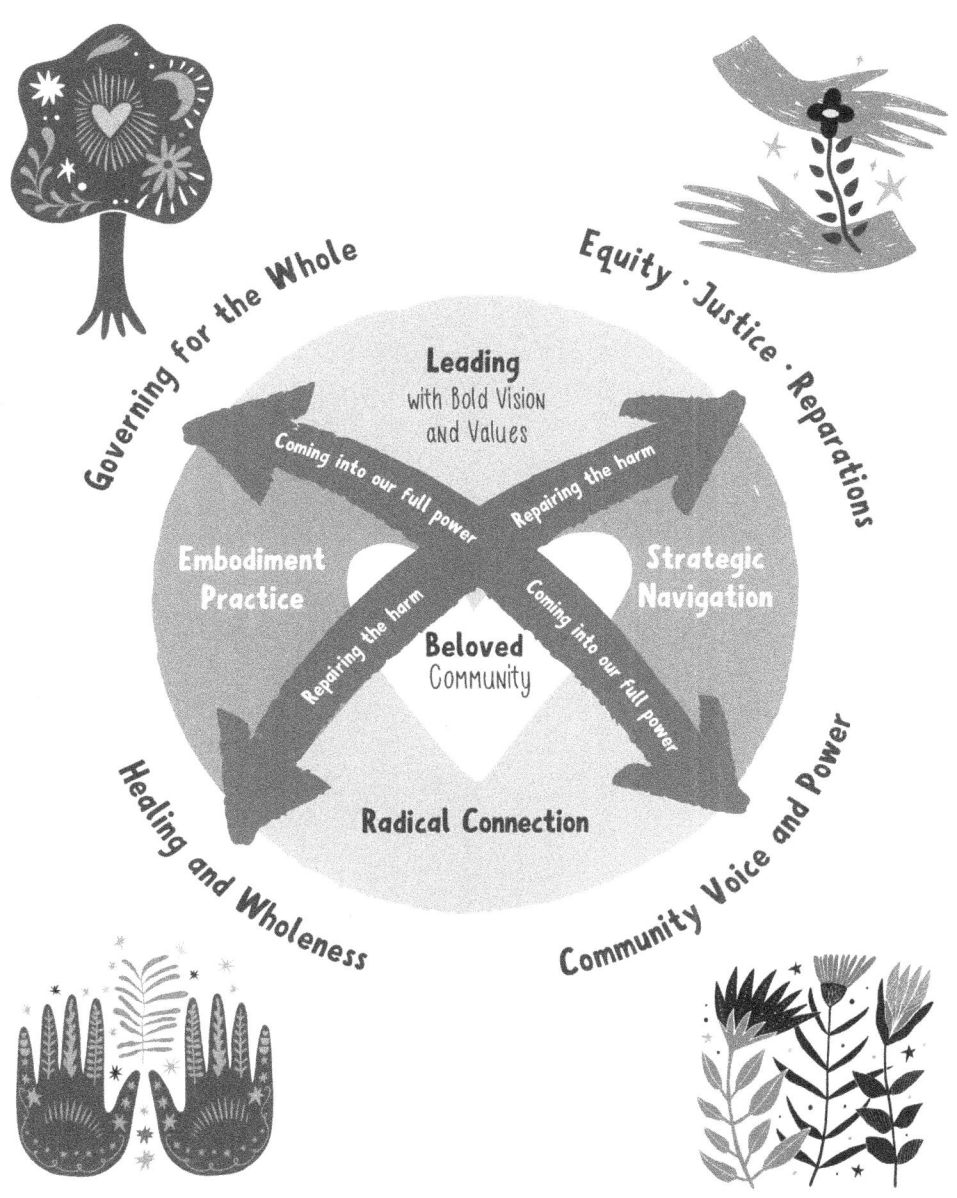

FOUR ELEMENTS AT THE CORE OF TRANSFORMATIVE MOVEMENT BUILDING

—BELOVED COMMUNITIES NETWORK

LEADING WITH BOLD vision and purpose, movement builders are moving beyond the question of "What do we need to do?" to ask, "Who do we need to be and what do we need to embody together to bring forth the transformation we seek?"

In this way, our movements are learning the art of time travel: starting by visioning the future we want, we are accelerating change by embodying and manifesting the values we seek in the world, right here and right now. We are not just asking people to believe another world is possible; we are inviting all of us to generate and experience a new world through *transformative practice* and strategy.

Beloved Communities Network recognizes four elements at the core of transformative movement building: leading with audacious *vision* and bold purpose; deeply *embodying* the values at the heart of the vision; building *radical connection* and deep community around the vision; and using all of that—vision, embodiment, and connection—to *strategically navigate* toward the future.

We are in the midst of the *Great Turning* and *Just Transition* from an extractive to a regenerative economy and a shift from a colonial worldview back to an Indigenous wisdom and worldview. *Transition practices* are the ways that help us to live and thrive and grow and heal in the midst of a polycrisis collapse of the old and reemergence of a "new-old world." *Just transition* is the practice of navigating contradictions"—*Movement Generation*. *Transition practice* supports us in drawing energy, resources, and legitimacy from forms of domination and shifting that energy toward reimagining and recreating the new.

Use the following chart to inspire hard conversations and soul-searching navigation for aligning your values and vision with your actions and strategy. This can become both a source of inspiration and a roadmap for your work. Take the concepts, qualities, and questions in this chart into your staff meetings, strategic planning, and discussions of short- and long-term aims for transformative changemaking. Returning to this chart over time can provide a north star in your group's clarification of your vision and purpose, how you embody it, how you deepen your connections to it and each other, and how all of this impacts your choices and strategies in the work.

What are the practices of transformative movements
that generate connection, community, and transformational resilience?

AUDACIOUS VISION	EMBODIMENT: Whole Person / Proactive Stance	RADICAL CONNECTION	STRATEGIC NAVIGATION
Transition practice recognizes that the future can guide us and that we are not constrained to the present or the past.	Transition practice recognizes that embodiment is crucial to ensuring that we have access to all the capacities we need.	Transition practice recognizes that everything gets done through relationships and nothing gets done without them.	Commitment to practice and action! The three foundational transition practices make strategic navigation possible.
Q: What do we want and how deeply do we want it?	Q: Who do we need to be to bring about the world we want and need? What do we need to consciously practice to be the people who reflect the vision?	Q: How are we connected? How do we honor our connections? Who is the "we"?	Q: How do we make choices that bring our whole selves and whole communities forward within changing and unpredictable conditions?
VISION AND COMMITMENT PRACTICES:	**EMBODIMENT PRACTICES:**	**RELATIONSHIP PRACTICES (MARGINS TO THE CENTER):**	**NAVIGATION PRACTICES:**
• Determining core purpose • Working toward wholeness • Shouldering courageous responsibility • Establishing a future narrative • Visualizing the long view	• Broadening awareness • Initiating a proactive stance • Generating and moving energy • Developing agility • Establishing rhythm • Expanding relational power • Nurturing creativity and play • Interrupting habits and redirecting	• Recognizing and reversing exclusion, isolation, and marginalization • Establishing radical connections and love • Building the "big we" and moving with those who are ready (small teams) • Recognizing interdependence • Recognizing/making space to heal from harm	• Following many paths up the mountain • Taking big leaps • Expanding networked action • Setting and resetting; learning as we go and adapting as we learn • Implementing decisiveness • Telling stories of navigation

Building Community
—BELOVED COMMUNITIES NETWORK

Organizing communities toward the vision that we seek to create requires us to build genuine relationships, trust, and accountability with folks that make up our collective. We must learn to rely on each other and expand our network of care to embrace each other. This activity allows participants to build deeper connections with each other. In pairs or small groups, discuss the following questions:

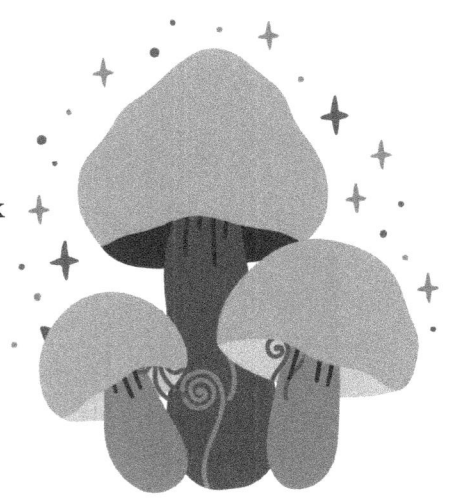

1. Who are your people, the people that you feel like you are walking or moving with toward a shared vision?

2. How have you felt cared for by community?

3. How have you cared for your community?

4. How do the values of this vision show up in your daily life and work together?

_____

_____

_____

What Is Your Shared Vision?   —BELOVED COMMUNITIES NETWORK

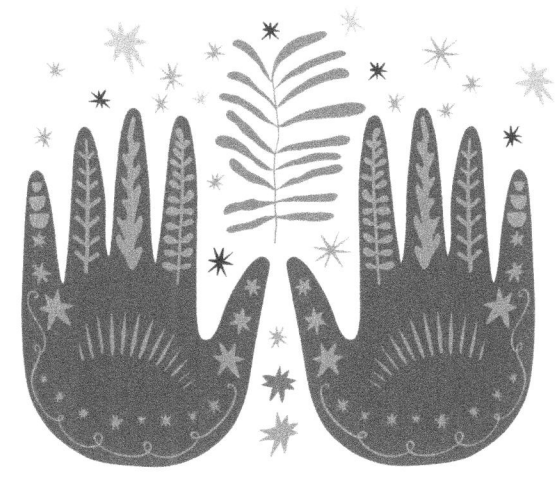

As an individual or as a group, think about your shared vision of the world one hundred years from now. The purpose of this activity is to enable you to integrate your dreams and desires of the world that you seek to create with others and to consider your role, your purpose, and your practices in navigating toward that vision. Transformative change has been happening for generations. We're building on the shoulders of our ancestors and we're trying to set things up for our descendants. We are not doing it alone and are a part of a collective of changemakers that contribute to the generational arc.

Take a few minutes to draw, doodle, or write about the future that you imagine for yourself, your family, your community, your organization, your nation, and the world. If you need more guidance, ask yourself what your work would look like seven generations from now. Envision what society would look like, smell like, and feel like.

"Future Stories" is an activity you can do that involves imagining a future descendant writing a letter of gratitude to their ancestors from one hundred years prior describing the future they are thriving in and what had to happen over those years for that reality to come into being. This includes describing the obstacles that were overcome and the key leaps, pivots, and breakthroughs that broke the cycle of incremental change and turned impossible challenges into inevitable victories. It is up to you to expand your imagination and the possibilities for this future.

FUTURE STORIES

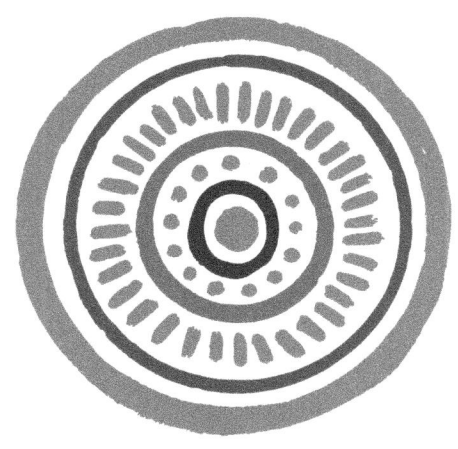

CREATIVE IMAGININGS

Innovation is crucial to being able to imagine a new way of being, yet creativity depends on our willingness and capacity to engage playfully and flexibly—that is, to throw away things we are familiar with and try something new, opening our visionary channels and unboxing ourselves from our associated thinking and conditioning. Often we've been educated out of creativity because the more we grow up, the more concerned we are that we might get things wrong, and that fear makes us more rigid, less willing to take risks and make mistakes, which in turn limits our creative freedom and innovation. Using our creativity to imagine new worlds into being resists these norms, while also facilitating connections and meaning-making with our fellow dreamers. This section encourages you to play, imagine, and create the world you want.

Collective Visioning Art Project —HALA KHOURI

For this exercise, you'll need a long table, a roll of art paper, water-soluble paint, paint brushes, cups of water to rinse brushes in, paper towels, and (optional) plastic gloves. It can be nice to play music as well to create a particular mood—preferably one that is creative and hopeful. To set up, roll out the art paper to whatever length your group requires so that everyone participating has a section to themselves. People should position themselves on one side of the table with paints and brushes available on the other side. Although paint is ideal, you can also do this with markers, crayons, and any type of art supplies. You can also set up on the ground if that is more accessible to folks. Feel free to get creative with the exercise![5]

INSTRUCTIONS:

1. Begin to paint something that represents your hope/vision for the work you are all doing together. Use images, colors, and words to express your vision, or consider making a collage. Don't be perfectionistic about this, and don't worry if it's not "good art."

2. If working in a group, make sure each person has room to paint their vision. After about fifteen minutes (you can determine the time), invite everyone to move over by one place (the person at the end of the table will have to move to the now-empty first spot at the table). Once everyone is at their new position, instruct them to add to the image started by the person next to them. Have them work on this for about five minutes and then switch again and again until everyone has contributed to each image.

3. When complete, invite folks to look at the final images and share their experience of the exercise. How did it feel to work alone and then add on layers of collaboration? How did the work change over time with different iterations of people's contributions? How could this be done differently? Who else would you invite to this vision work?

4. You can keep the mural intact or cut it up into pieces and give a piece to each participant.

5. In future iterations, you can return to the mural and discuss action steps to actualize the visions therein.

Human Sculpture —ADAPTED FROM AUGUSTO BOAL[6]

This is a collaborative group exercise that invites people to explore the goals of their work together in an embodied and creative way. This process can shed light on different dynamics that will naturally emerge in various efforts aimed at making change to the status quo. This is important because sometimes difficult situations can be a sign of growth and positive change, so anticipating and understanding this can allow for a stronger collaboration and ability to withstand the difficult parts of change work.

1. As a group, come up with a list of words, phrases, or sentences that describe the goals of your organization or endeavors and the problem(s) it seeks to solve (examples: to contribute toward a world where all workers are treated fairly and

are given humane conditions to work in; to change systems of oppression and create new liberatory systems of collaboration and mutual care).

2. Have a group of people volunteer to create a human sculpture representing the current condition of things you wish to change. This human sculpture will represent the situation that the organization is addressing, as identified in step 1 (i.e., inhumane working conditions where workers don't have rights). This can be done with between three and twelve people.

3. If there are people observing, invite them to each come and make one change to the sculpture to move it in the direction of the shared goal that was identified in step 1. This could mean having one person change their stance, or another person move where they are positioned, and so on. Each person makes one change until they feel the sculpture now represents their shared goal. (People can also step out from the sculpture to suggest changes.)

4. Keep reminding people to notice how they feel in their body at each stage. How does embodying the goals of the work change your relationship to it or understanding of it?

5. At the end, discuss what that process was like and what it might reveal to them about their work together. Return to the goals stated in step 1 to see if new insights about the goal itself or how to achieve it have emerged through this collective embodiment practice.

MOBIUS LIVING AGREEMENTS

OUR LIBERATORY TECH colleagues Sará King and Davion "Zi" Ziere have shared a beautiful statement of how their organization wants to build, dream, and work together through healing-in-action liberatory transformations. Their agreements might be adaptable to you and those you work, play, and dream with.

Healing, Justice, and Equity: Living in a culture of domination means that we have a lot of healing to do from the ways we have been harmed by white supremacy, patriarchy, capitalism, and heteronormativity. We conscientiously explore what it means to heal ourselves, to prioritize individual and collective well-being, to redistribute power among ourselves, and to continually develop an understanding of what it means to show up with integrity to these principles. We practice embodying these qualities because they live in, and are expressed through, the body.

Spirit Is an Integral Force: We hold that Spirit is present in however we wish to connect to and honor that which is greater than ourselves. Spirit is a collaborative force behind everything that we do. A person can make meaning of connecting with Spirit in many ways, and we affirm the vast diversity of people's experiences.

Wholeness and Embodiment: In contrast to the dominant culture's emphasis on the thinking mind, we honor the whole person and the wisdom held in the body. We believe that slowing down to notice sensation enables us to avoid harm and promote healing.

Acknowledge Trauma and Emotions: All bodies carry stress and a legacy of intergenerational trauma. Emotions are one of the primary means by which we express what has meaning to us, how we wish to be seen, and what we need from those around us. Emotional reactivity is a normal result of stress and the pressure to "perform" or "produce," especially in organizational contexts. At Mobius, we recognize that it is very important to create a safe and brave space where people can have their emotions and/or trauma recognized when they arise. By slowing down and naming what is arising, we can intentionally practice cultivating presence. This allows us to see and hear one another more fully and supports our holistic well-being.

Emergence and Engagement with Time: "Emergence is the way complex systems and patterns arise out of a multiplicity of relatively simple interactions."[7] In order to notice these patterns and cocreate with each other and with Spirit, we honor emergence. This requires us to hold relationships with time differently: some meetings require more fluidity and spaciousness while others need to be time fixed. And doing all of this requires a good dose of grace and humor.[8]

What might your living agreements be in your collaboration or organization?

LIVING AGREEMENTS

When/What/Why/Where/Who Exercise   —HALA KHOURI

Use the next few pages to envision how you might use the ideas and practices in this book.

Name the practices you want to use and then have each member of your group answer the questions for each practice. The following space allows you to envision this for several situations/scenarios in which you'd use different practices from the book.

SCENARIO #1: PRACTICE NAME AND PAGE NUMBER:

_____

When: What is the circumstance or time when you could use this practice?

_____

_____

_____

What: What supplies, skills, structure, and support might be needed to do it well?

_____

_____

_____

Why: What is the intention and goal of facilitating this practice?

_____

_____

_____

Where: Where are all the places you can imagine using this?

_____

_____

_____

Who: Who is the best person to facilitate this? Who do you want to invite to participate?

_____

_____

_____

SCENARIO #2: PRACTICE NAME AND PAGE NUMBER:

_____

When: What is the circumstance or time when you could use this practice?

_____

_____

_____

What: What supplies, skills, structure, and support might be needed to do it well?

_____

_____

_____

Why: What is the intention and goal of facilitating this practice?

_____

_____

_____

Where: Where are all the places you can imagine using this?

_____

_____

_____

Who: Who is the best person to facilitate this? Who do you want to invite to participate?

_____

_____

_____

SCENARIO #3: PRACTICE NAME AND PAGE NUMBER:

_____

When: What is the circumstance or time when you could use this practice?

_____

_____

_____

What: What supplies, skills, structure, and support might be needed to do it well?

Why: What is the intention and goal of facilitating this practice?

Where: Where are all the places you can imagine using this?

Who: Who is the best person to facilitate this? Who do you want to invite to participate?

CLOSING THOUGHTS

Healing is the work of both resistance and affirmation. We are showing up to learn how to take care of ourselves and our communities, repair harm, restore relationships, create radical visions for change, and build the infrastructures and safety nets we need to do so. These small practices of healing, community building, and personal transformation will invariably have a rippling effect on a larger level. Through this effort, we are doing the work of creating spaces, practices, and conditions to ensure that radical care and healing take place for individual changemakers and collectives, organizations, and institutions of changemaking.

It often feels impossible to pause and reflect on our well-being and hopes for a better world in moments when the stakes are so high, but as Bayo Akomolafe reminds us, "the times are urgent, let us slow down."[9] Let us choose right here and now to (re)claim a moment of rest and community care to cultivate well-being and liberation in mind, body, heart, and spirit, individually and collectively. Let us move forward from a place of broken systems toward bringing healing, joy, emotional intimacy, openness, and our whole selves into communities, organizations, and movements for peace and justice. Let us deepen our relationship with ourselves, our ancestors, and each other through authentic interconnectedness. Let us embrace a calling to heal the root causes of pain, to be the change we are wanting, and to build new systems of political, social, economic, and cultural care for our families, communities, and the next generation. Let us choose this in our hearts, in our actions, and in our collective work, again and again.

As you have joined us on this journey and worked through this workbook, we hope it has become more of a *play*book, a work of art, a journal, or a place for contemplative healing, support, and inspiration. We encourage you to keep trying out these practices alone, with friends, in ceremony, in nature, and at work; reflect on the ideas and manifest practices of your own that transform concept into action. One by one, community by community, movement by movement, this fractal will ripple outward until we have a mass of healing justice practices informing our collective transformation toward well-being, social change, and liberation.

HELPFUL RESOURCES

Follow these links to learn more knowledge, tools, and practices and to connect with the contributors of this workbook and those who directly influence our work:

- *American Detox*: Kerri Kelly: www.americandetox.co/about
- Beloved Communities Network: www.belovedcommunitiesnetwork.org
- Booker: www.lesliebooker.com
- CASA Pitzer: www.pitzer.edu/casa-pitzer/pitzer-ontario/events/know-justice -know-peace
- Emergent Strategy Ideation Institute: www.esii.org
- Generative Somatics: www.generativesomatics.org/resources
- The Haize Way: Haize Hawke: www.haizehawke.com
- Hala Khouri: www.halakhouri.com
- Jacoby Ballard Yoga: www.jacobyballard.net
- Lumos Transforms: www.lumostransforms.com
- Mobius: www.mobi.us.org
- Move to End Violence: www.movetoendviolence.org/resources
- Movement Strategy Center: www.movementstrategy.org/msc-resources
- Partnership for Safety and Justice: www.safetyandjustice.org
- Pedagogy and Theater of the Oppressed: www.ptoweb.org
- Susy Zepeda: www.chi.ucdavis.edu/people/susy-zepeda
- Tessa Hicks Peterson: www.tessahickspeterson.com

CONTRIBUTORS

Jacoby Ballard   Jacoby is a trans social justice educator and yoga teacher who leads workshops and trainings around the country on diversity, equity, and inclusion, with a focus at the nexus of healing and social justice. More of his teachings can be found on his website and in his book, *A Queer Dharma: Yoga and Meditations for Liberation.*

Beloved Communities Network   Beloved Communities Network collaborates with a network of partners that are transitioning to a world of love, interdependence, and resilience, guided by a holistic approach that includes leading with bold vision and values, embodied practice, radical connection, and strategic navigation. More of their teachings can be found in the resources section of their website.

Leslie Booker   Leslie brings her heart and wisdom to the intersection of Dharma, Embodied Wisdom, and liberation. Using this framework, through her teaching and writing on changing the paradigm of self and community care, she supports folks in creating a culture of belonging. She shares her offerings widely as a university lecturer, public speaker, and Buddhist philosophy and meditation teacher. Leslie is passionate about supporting frontline communities to thrive in their work. She currently lives in Philadelphia with her partner and pup and serves as the guiding teacher of New York Insight. More of her teachings can be found on her website.

Scarlett Duarte   Scarlett is an Afro-Indigenous, Two-Spirit, Black abolitionist feminist and frontline organizer with a passion for creating transformative community connections and building power to collectively end systems of injustice. She brings her direct life experiences with trauma, violence, grief, sobriety, and grassroots social justice organizing to the intersection with traditional ancestral medicine and reclamation and reconnection with the ancestors. More of her work can be explored by contacting her directly through the CASA Pitzer website.

Kazu Haga   Kazu is a trainer, advocate, and practitioner of nonviolence, restorative justice, and mindfulness. He works to support healing for individuals, collectives, and societies by combining various organizing and healing modalities, working in prisons and jails, high schools and youth groups, and with activist communities around the country. More of his teachings can be found in his book *Healing Resistance: A Radically Different Response to Harm.*

Haize Hawke   Haize is a spiritual counselor, mentor, healer, master doula, and world traveler. Haize facilitates how to live a heart-led life and be midwives and doulas to the new consciousness and action we need today for personal healing and collective justice. More of her teachings can be found on her website and in her program: "Get Rooted Doula Training: The Haize Way."

Kerri Kelly   Kerri is the founder of CTZNWELL, a movement that is democratizing well-being for all. A descendant of generations of firemen and first responders, Kerri has dedicated her life to kicking down doors and fighting for justice. She's been teaching yoga for over twenty years and is known for making waves in the wellness industry by challenging norms, disrupting systems, and mobilizing people to act. More of her teachings can be found on her website and in her book, *American Detox: The Myth of Wellness and How We Can Truly Heal.*

Hala Khouri   Hala Khouri has been teaching yoga and movement for over twenty-five years and has been doing clinical work and trainings for fifteen years. Originally from Beirut, Lebanon, Hala has dedicated her life to the work of trauma-informed care, embodied social justice, trauma-informed education, and resilience. She cofounded Off the Mat, Into the World, a training organization to bridge yoga and activism within a social justice framework, and she leads Collective Resilience trauma-informed yoga and somatics trainings nationally. More of her teachings can be found on her website and in her book, *Peace from Anxiety: Get Grounded, Build Resilience and Stay Connected Amidst the Chaos.*

Mobius   Mobius is a home for people creating Liberatory Technology products, systems, and narratives. Their mission is to activate and support a tech ecosystem focused on healing and liberation, prioritizing Black, Brown, Indigenous, queer people, youth, and others who are marginalized by the dominant tech sector. Mobius weaves together a supportive community of people who are building and enabling Liberatory Technology, including regenerative investors, scholars, storytellers, and non-fellow technologists, entrepreneurs, and artists.

Keely Nguyễn   Keely Nguyễn comes from a legacy of strong-willed women in rural/coastal provinces of Southern Vietnam. As a first-generation Vietnamese American from a working-class background, Keely is passionate about sharing collective memories and cultural stories to resist and build community with folks, specifically directly impacted youth. She currently works as a communications manager at Partnership for Safety and Justice, working to disrupt the carceral state through narrative building, advocacy, and digital organizing. More information can be found through that organization's website.

Tessa Hicks Peterson   Tessa was raised in a family of activists, artists, and teachers in the eclectic community of Venice Beach, which has informed her work spanning twenty-five years with civil rights and social justice nonprofits and in higher education. She has directed a number of community centers, facilitated hundreds of workshops, and taught classes at Pitzer College in anti-bias education, movement arts, healing justice, and community-based research collaborations. More of her teachings can be found on her website and in her books, *Student Development and Social Justice: Critical Learning, Radical Healing, and Community Engagement* and *Liberating the Classroom: Healing and Justice in Higher Education.*

Susy Zepeda   Susy is a transdisciplinary, decolonial feminist and community-centered scholar, teacher, and practitioner with a focus on Xicana Indígena spirit work. Her work is rooted in decolonization, critical feminist of color collaborative methodologies, oral and visual storytelling, and intergenerational healing. More of her teachings can be found in her 2022 book, *Queering Mesoamerican Diasporas: Remembering Xicana Indígena Ancestries.*

NOTES

Introduction

1 The *Practicing Liberation* anthology grew out of the work of the Know Justice, Know Peace Community Collective, a transformation and justice project that includes community-based action research, organizational and personal development workshops, and ongoing coaching and community building around healing justice, facilitated by CASA Pitzer with six local community-based organizations in Southern California's Inland Region. Details about that project and expanded explorations of healing justice can be found in the anthology. Portions of this workbook have been adapted from the anthology (Peterson and Khouri, *Practicing Liberation*) as well as the editors' other books including Khouri's *Peace from Anxiety* and Peterson's *Student Development and Social Justice* and *Liberating the Classroom: Healing and Justice in Higher Education*. (2025)

Part I

1 Practices from Hala Khouri were created specifically for this workbook or adapted from Khouri, *Peace from Anxiety*.
2 Sugawara et al., "Effects of Interoceptive Training."
3 This quote is from Valorie Thomas's "breath. fugitivity. wild horses: Black Feminist Strategies for Healing in a Predatory Empire" in Peterson and Khouri, *Practicing Liberation*.
4 Hạnh, *Creating True Peace*, 59.
5 Yerkes and Dodson, "Strength of Stimulus to Rapidity of Habit-Formation," 459–82.
6 Levine, *Waking the Tiger*.
7 Chuang-Tzu is credited with the famous Chinese Buddhist saying "When you open your heart, you get life's ten thousand sorrows, and ten thousand joys."
8 Jampolsky, *Letting Go of Fear*.
9 I learned this meditation practice from Eric Kolvig during early LGBTQ meditation retreats of the 1990s in the Insight tradition. The fourth direction was added by Larry Yang.
10 Boorstein, *"Let's See What Happens Next."*
11 Freire, *Pedagogy of the Oppressed*.
12 For those desiring more knowledge about the roots and manifestations of the rapidly growing healing justice movement, we recommend reading Page and Woodland, *Healing Justice Lineages*.
13 Freire, *Pedagogy of the Oppressed*.
14 Kelly, *American Detox*.
15 Adapted from Peterson, *Student Development and Social Justice*, 199.
16 This exercise has been adapted from Theatre of the Oppressed; more can be found in the founder's seminal book: Boal, *Theatre of the Oppressed*.

Part II

1 West, "Justice is what love looks like in public."
2 Adapted from Peterson, *Student Development and Social Justice*, 399.
3 This exercise has been adapted from Boal, *Theatre of the Oppressed*. More information can be found there.
4 Adapted from Peterson, *Student Development and Social Justice*, 377.
5 Adapted from Peterson, *Student Development and Social Justice*, 379.
6 For further resources that explore topics of transformative leadership, we encourage you to look into some of our favorites: Brown, *Dare to Lead*; LeBlanc, *Broken: How Our Social Systems Are Failing Us*; Center for Courage and Renewal and Francis, *The Courage Way*; Wheatley, *Finding Our Way*; and Eller and Hierck, *Trauma-Sensitive Leadership*.

Part III

1 Kelley, *Freedom Dreams*.
2 Adapted from Nkem Ndefo, "Micro to Macro: Embodied Trauma-Informed and Resilience-Oriented Systems Change," in Peterson and Khouri, *Practicing Liberation*.
3 Much of this introductory section has been adapted from Peterson, *Liberating the Classroom*.
4 This framework and correlating questions have been adapted from Baghai, Coley, and White, *The Alchemy of Growth*; Raworth, "Three Horizons"; and Peterson, *Liberating the Classroom*.
5 This exercise has been adapted from one shared by Liza Auciello.
6 This exercise came from Boal, *Theatre of the Oppressed*. More information can be found there.
7 brown, *Emergent Strategy*, 6.
8 Davis and King, "Living Agreements."
9 Akomolafe and Benavides, "The Times Are Urgent."

BIBLIOGRAPHY

Akomolafe, Bayo, and Marta Benavides. "The Times Are Urgent: Let's Slow Down." Accessed October 6, 2023. https://www.bayoakomolafe.net/post/the-times-are-urgent-lets-slow-down.

Baghai, Mehrdad, Steve Coley, and David White. *The Alchemy of Growth: Practical Insights for Building the Enduring Enterprise*. New York: Basic Books, 1999.

Boal, Augusto. *Theatre of the Oppressed*. New York: Theatre Communications Group, 1993.

Boorstein, Sylvia. "Let's See What Happens Next." *Sylvia Boorstein* (blog). November 7, 2016. https://www.sylviaboorstein.com/?offset=1483242955090.

brown, adrienne maree. *Emergent Strategy: Shaping Change, Changing Worlds*. Chico, CA: AK Press, 2017.

Brown, Brené. *Dare to Lead: Brave Work. Tough Conversations. Whole Hearts*. New York: Random House, 2018.

Center for Courage and Renewal and Shelly L. Francis. *The Courage Way: Leading and Living with Integrity*. Oakland, CA: Berrett-Koehler, 2018.

Davis, Julia Rhodes, and Sará King. "Living Agreements: Creating the Conditions for Our Co-Liberation," *Medium*. April 1, 2022. https://medium.com/@mobiusorg/living-agreements-creating-the-conditions-for-our-co-liberation-8acba1dea439.

Eller, John F., and Tom Hierck. *Trauma-Sensitive Leadership: Creating a Safe and Predictable School Environment*. Bloomington, IN: Solution Tree Press, 2022.

Freire, Paulo. *Pedagogy of the Oppressed*, 30th Anniversary ed. Translated by Myra Bergman Ramos. New York: Continuum, 2000.

Hạnh, Thích Nhất. *Creating True Peace: Ending Violence in Yourself, Your Family, Your Community, and the World*. New York: Atria Books, 2003.

Hạnh, Thích Nhất. *Peace Is Every Step: The Path of Mindfulness in Everyday Life*. New York: Bantam Books, 1991.

Jampolsky, Gerald. *Letting Go of Fear*. New York: Bantam, 1979.

Kelley, Robin D. G. *Freedom Dreams: The Black Radical Imagination*. Boston: Beacon Press, 2022.

Kelly, Kerri. *American Detox: The Myth of Wellness and How We Can Truly Heal*. Berkeley, CA: North Atlantic Books, 2022.

Khouri, Hala. *Peace from Anxiety: Get Grounded, Build Resilience and Stay Connected Amidst the Chaos*. Boulder, CO: Shambhala Publications, 2021.

LeBlanc, Paul. *Broken: How Our Social Systems Are Failing Us and How We Can Fix Them*. Dallas: Matt Holt Books, an imprint of BenBella Books, 2022.

Levine, Peter. *Waking the Tiger: Healing Trauma*. Berkeley, CA: North Atlantic Books, 1997.

Page, Cara, and Erica Woodland. *Healing Justice Lineages: Dreaming at the Crossroads of Liberation, Collective Care, and Safety*. Berkeley, CA: North Atlantic Books, 2023.

Peterson, Tessa Hicks. *Liberating the Classroom: Healing and Justice in Higher Education*. Baltimore: Johns Hopkins University Press, forthcoming 2025.

Peterson, Tessa Hicks. *Student Development and Social Justice: Critical Learning, Radical Healing, and Community Engagement.* New York: Palgrave Macmillan, 2017.

Peterson, Tessa Hicks, and Hala Khouri, eds. *Practicing Liberation: Transformative Strategies for Collective Healing and Systems Change.* Berkeley, CA: North Atlantic Books, 2024.

Raworth, Kate. "Three Horizons Framework—A Quick Introduction" (YouTube). *Doughnut Economics Action Lab.* August 8, 2018. https://youtu.be/_5KfRQJqpPU?si=_yrPZPp6YIa_895D.

Sugawara, Ayako, Yuri Terasawa, Ruri Katsunuma, and Atsushi Sekiguchi. "Effects of Interoceptive Training on Decision Making, Anxiety, and Somatic Symptoms." *Biopsychosocial Medicine* 14, no. 1 (March 2020): 1–8. https://doi.org/10.1186/s13030-020-00179-7.

West, Cornel. "Justice is what love looks like in public. Tenderness is what love feels like in private." Speaking at an Askwith Education Forum at Harvard Graduate School of Education (Facebook video). October 24, 2017.

Wheatley, Margaret J. *Finding Our Way: Leadership for an Uncertain Time.* San Francisco: Berrett-Koehler, 2007.

Yerkes, Robert, and John Dodson. "The Relation of Strength of Stimulus to Rapidity of Habit-Formation." *Journal of Comparative Neurology and Psychology* 18 (1908): 459–82.

ABOUT NORTH ATLANTIC BOOKS

North Atlantic Books (NAB) is an independent, nonprofit publisher committed to a bold exploration of the relationships between mind, body, spirit, and nature. Founded in 1974, NAB aims to nurture a holistic view of the arts, sciences, humanities, and healing. To make a donation or to learn more about our books, authors, events, and newsletter, please visit www.northatlanticbooks.com.

01 14